A Loving Approach to Dementia Care

A 36-Hour Day Book

A Loving Approach to Dementia Care

Making Meaningful Connections
with the Person Who Has Alzheimer's Disease
or Other Dementia or Memory Loss

SECOND EDITION

LAURA WAYMAN

Johns Hopkins University Press
Baltimore

Johns Hopkins University Press
2715 North Charles Street
Baltimore, Maryland 21218-4363
www.press.jhu.edu

Library of Congress Cataloging-in-Publication Data

Names: Wayman, Laura, 1955– author.
Title: A loving approach to dementia care : making meaningful connections with the person who has Alzheimer's disease or other dementia or memory loss / Laura Wayman.
Description: Second edition. | Baltimore : Johns Hopkins University Press, [2017] | Includes bibliographical references and index.
Identifiers: LCCN 2016035400 | ISBN 9781421422282 (pbk. : alk. paper) | ISBN 142142228X (pbk. : alk. paper) | ISBN 9781421422299 (electronic) | ISBN 1421422298 (electronic)
Subjects: LCSH: Dementia—Patients—Care—Popular works. | Alzheimer's disease—Patients—Care—Popular works.
Classification: LCC RC521 .W39 2017 | DDC 616.8/3—dc23
LC record available at https://lccn.loc.gov/2016035400

A catalog record for this book is available from the British Library.

Special discounts are available for bulk purchases of this book. For more information, please contact Special Sales at 410-516-6936 or specialsales@press.jhu.edu.

Johns Hopkins University Press uses environmentally friendly book materials, including recycled text paper that is composed of at least 30 percent post-consumer waste, whenever possible.

CONTENTS

FOREWORD

CARY G. ROTTER, *Memphis Comfort Keepers*

In this book Laura Wayman presents a ground-breaking new approach to dementia care that encompasses everything from understanding what the condition is (and is not) to its implications for those who suffer with it and their caregivers. Much has been written about dementia disorders, from diagnosis to treatment to tools for caregivers; it is Laura's unique methodology and perspective that make her insights so valuable to families struggling with dementia care and its implications.

A Loving Approach to Dementia Care is written with compassion and understanding for the caregivers who frequently sacrifice their own health in caring for a loved one. Laura's methodology is refreshingly different and accessible because of its simplicity and practicality; it is not the clinician who speaks to us from an academic viewpoint but the practitioner whose strategies have been borne out in facility settings and thousands of individual homes across the country. As a daughter who experienced firsthand the pernicious impact of Alzheimer's on both the sufferer (her father) and his caregiver (her mother), Laura writes with the passion of conviction and proven experience.

Science struggles with most dementia disorders, especially Alzheimer's, because treatment options are limited. The formulaic approach to dealing with these disorders rarely broaches the real-life challenges of caregivers grappling with a landscape that changes ruthlessly and frequently. Most caregivers seek to learn a path to help them navigate each day. But unfortunately what works for short periods does not work indefinitely. As Laura explains, caregivers must embrace the present and live in the moment.

This book is all about moments. Countless moments, day in and day out; moments of wonder, exasperation, tears, triumphs, mistakes, learning experiences, and spiritual challenge. But it is also a book of hope and love and sacrifice through which we enhance meaning in our lives as we learn more about who we are when caregiving becomes our role or calling.

Laura is our guide in a universe as topsy-turvy as *Alice in Wonderland* and inverted as *The Twilight Zone*. Caregivers will be relieved to discover virtually every situation they encounter is addressed in some fashion, with one caveat. As Laura explains, dementia cases are as singular as fingerprints. As no two cases are identical, approaches must be tweaked. But caregivers reading this book will discover solutions that work and are flexible in application. Importantly, Laura distills the rationale behind her approaches in such clear and logical fashion that caregivers will learn to refine and trust their instincts when new challenges arise.

In this second edition of *A Loving Approach to Dementia Care* Laura has added two new chapters that expand the spectrum of caregiving from the individual to entire communities. Chapter three addresses the typical first response of a dementia diagnosis, which is denial. Denial ultimately evolves to acceptance—but only after the preponderance of evidence is overwhelming. If dementia acceptance is inevitable for any objective caregiver presented with its telltale signs and timeline, and given the avalanche of dementia disorders we are facing as a society, then why should community acceptance not be the logical extension?

Also new to this edition is chapter four, which deals with anosognosia. This biological condition precludes our ability to even be aware of the existence of illness. Is anosognosia perhaps analogous to society's slowness in becoming dementia-aware at a macro level and facilitating appropriate community responses to what is becoming a pandemic?

Laura Wayman's book is a clarion call to action—positive, life-affirming, constructive action that helps us better cope with a condition whose boundaries for now are essentially out of our control. There is an analogue in Laura's call to arms to Viktor Frankl's *Man's Search for Meaning*. Frankl asserted that ultimately each individual remains entirely unfettered in interpreting actions and circumstances beyond his or her control in a manner that allows the individual to transcend the oppression of an implacable foe. We too have that freedom and responsibility in combating dementia disorders. Laura gives us the tools and inspiration to fight a battle where loss is not the inevitable outcome. Individually and collectively, we would be wise to pay heed to Laura's message.

THANKS AND APPRECIATION

I thank my husband, Stephen Wayman, for his patience and support. (Boy, did he have a lot of it!) He has steadfastly continued to be my pillar of light, my fountain of love, and a constant source of comfort along the second leg of this amazing journey.

To my daughter Alicia, for her contributions as a supporting author and encourager. To my daughter Angie, who was always the long-distance promoter, cheering me on from afar. And to all of my family, who have been there for me all along the way.

To those who have continued to support me through the long birthing process (including this second time around!): DanaLyn Brophy, Deanna Chitambar, Rachel Cline, Scott and Faye Cluthe, Teri Crocker, Pamela Dallas, Denise Davis, Joe Dunham, Lisa Emmerling, Dr. Barbara Gillogly, Cindy Gustafson, Jocelyn Kaufenberg, Gerrie Kuster, Vince Maffeo, Cary and Wendy Rotter, Rob Stewart, and Caren Terry.

A special thanks to Phillip and Taryn Benson of Bensonwrites, whose expert editing and copywriting made this book flow and come together with beauty and grace. Their kind words, professionalism, and conviction gave me the strength to make it to the finish line.

I want to express my heartfelt appreciation for the warm and supportive response I have received as a new, as well as a second edition, author from everyone at Johns Hopkins University Press in readying my work to be presented to the world. From day one, getting communication and guidance from Jacqueline Wehmueller, Executive Editor, has been an overall positive experience way beyond what "thank you" can express. And the entire JHUP "team" has worked, and continues to work, tirelessly with me, all the while presenting profound consideration, understanding, and professional commitment. Truly you all are a shining example of the gold standard in customer service, showing Johns Hopkins University Press as the leader and innovator in scholarly publishing worldwide.

And to my dear friends who held my hand and whispered the necessary nurturing encouragement: Alan and Denise Pedersen and Cindy Gustafson.

To all the caregivers who honored me with their stories, struggles, strength, moments of success, and commitment.

And a very sincere thank you to the countless people who initiated this book by asking me, "Do you have a book?" (and more recently with the question I am often asked, "When can we read your second edition?").

This book is dedicated to the loving memory of my mother.

A Loving Approach to Dementia Care

CHAPTER ONE

Introduction

Navigating the Journey

Caring for a person who has dementia is a labor of devotion and patience. Sadly, many caregivers selflessly sacrifice their own well-being during the process. In addition, many caregivers, whether they are lay caregivers looking after a loved one at home or professionals working in a clinical setting, do not have the knowledge or training they need to meet the challenges of dementia. That is exactly where successful caregiving breaks down.

Providing care is an important and noble endeavor, but to be able to provide the best possible care, you must also take care of *yourself.* So pause here and ask yourself one simple question: would it be okay with you, the caregiver, if you experienced a lasting sense of relief?

I have asked many caregivers this question.

Not surprisingly, not one has answered "No."

If you are caring for someone with a form of dementia (such as Alzheimer's disease) or another cognitive impairment, this book is intended to help lighten your load every day. It is possible to simultaneously provide better care both for the person with dementia and for yourself.

Of course, every family and situation is different. You may have been thrust into this caregiving role unexpectedly—without any training or even any encouragement. Perhaps the care is being provided at home, with or without other family or professional in-home support.

Or maybe the care is provided in a specialized memory care unit, an assisted living environment, or a skilled nursing facility. Although caregiving is often inspiring and rewarding, it can be very difficult. Caring for someone with a cognitive impairment can be even more difficult than caring for someone with a physical impairment who is fully competent mentally and emotionally. The complications of confusion, forgetfulness, and memory loss, and the behaviors that go along with them, can be traumatic for the person with the disease and for the person providing care. Because of the dementia, neither the person involved nor the relationship will ever be the same.

Along with the challenges of caring for a person who has a form of dementia, caregivers—especially family members—will experience conflicting emotions. Their feelings may swing from guilt, denial, and distress one moment to empathy, acceptance, and understanding the next. Not every circumstance is happy, positive, or easy. You may only rarely come to a place of acceptance or understanding about this experience, or maybe not at all. You may struggle to find any meaning along the road you are traveling.

During my decades of working with caregivers, I have heard many accounts of what the experience is like—from the sad and hollow to experiences rich in significance. Everyone faces obstacles when caring for a loved one; some of these obstacles come in the form of uncomfortable or painful emotional histories or past unresolved conflicts. Yet with an open mind, you can essentially "feel your way" through the process, taking a more holistic view of your unique dementia-care circumstances and challenges. The following popular fable gently illustrates how each person's perception of dementia, however different it may be from someone else's experience, is nevertheless "right."

The Elephant and the Blind Men

Once upon a time, there lived six blind men in a village. One day, the villagers told them, "Hey, there is an elephant in the village today."

They had no idea what an elephant was. They decided, "Even though we would not be able to see it, let us go and feel it." All of them went to the elephant. Every one of them touched the elephant.

"Hey, the elephant is like a pillar," said the first man, who touched the leg of the elephant.

"Oh, no! It is like a rope," said the second man, who touched the tail.

"Oh, no! It is like a thick branch of a tree," said the third man, who touched the elephant's trunk.

"It is like a big hand fan," said the fourth man, who touched the ear.

"It is like a huge wall," said the fifth man, who touched the belly.

"It is like a solid pipe," said the sixth man, who touched the tusk.

The men began to argue about the elephant, and every one of them insisted that he was "right." A wise man was passing by. He stopped and asked them what was the matter.

"We cannot agree on what the elephant is like," they told him.

And the wise man calmly explained: "All of you are right. Each one of you has a different idea because each of you touched a different part of the elephant. So, actually, the elephant has all of those features—everything you all said."

That ended the argument. They all were happy that they all were "right."

Anekantvad, or *The Theory of Manifold Predictions*

I originally read this fable when I was young. At the time, I was amused by the poor blind man who had to feel the tail. Of course, there could be serious implications with that particular anatomical end of an elephant. Years later, I know that as a caregiver, you may feel as if you are living out a more contemporary proverb: "Some days you're the pigeon, and some days you're the statue."

Your loved one (or client or resident, if you are a professional caregiver) may have a variety of challenges that stem from physical, emotional, and behavioral causes. Perhaps the person you are caring for is unable to communicate clearly without crying, due to a brain injury that diminished his or her ability to control sad or painful emotions. You may be caring for a parent who was verbally or even physically abusive to you or who did not make you feel safe and loved as a child. Now you are attempting to develop a new relationship, even though you cannot erase your feelings or memories. As a result of these and many other factors, you are touching only part of the dementia "elephant," able to view only part of the situation that the dementia has inserted into your life.

I have spent many years assisting caregivers just like you. As you read about the diverse experiences that I and others have had working with dementia-challenged adults, their families, and professional caregivers, you will gain more insight into the intriguing world where the adult with dementia exists. You will also develop a new perspective on many of the common obstacles facing care providers and learn to enjoy your loved one or client at a deeper level. This book—and the special techniques described within it—will equip you with the compass you need to navigate this journey successfully.

Caregivers frequently ask for the "right way" to respond to the difficult behaviors they encounter. While there is no one-size-fits-all magic formula, there are many proven techniques to help guide you. My personal studies in this field have included excellent foundational resources, such as *The Validation Breakthrough*, by Naomi Feil; *The 36-Hour Day*, by Nancy L. Mace and Peter V. Rabins; and *The Best Friend's Approach to Alzheimer's Care*, by Virginia Bell and David Troxel.

My vision is to share as much knowledge and insight with you as possible, both from my own experiences and from those of other professional and family caregivers. Each chapter chronicles a real-life story about caregiving. You may very well find yourself relating to these heartwarming accounts. Every story is followed by two sections, "Lessons Learned" and "Perceptions and Approaches," that can empower you and make your situation more manageable. Use these tools to make traveling this frequently arduous trek much less stressful and much more successful.

In the chapters of this book I describe the *affirmative response method of communication*. This communication style is based on the insight that it is impossible to bring adults with dementia "into reality." Instead of attempting to correct the dementia-challenged person's perception of the world, you can learn to affirm your loved one or client's view of reality and to relate to him or her within that framework. As you give affirmative responses to the dementia-challenged person, you will receive the same from him or her in return, confirming that you have successfully made a connection.

The affirmative response method uses simple and valuable techniques to facilitate quality interactions and enhanced emotional connections with the person who has dementia. These interactions and communications reduce the caregiver's stress level. This innovative approach to communicating opens a window into the world where your loved one or client exists. It will increase your awareness of the equally important need for your own care and the vital role you play in the caregiver–care receiver relationship.

As I travel the country supporting, training, and encouraging caregivers on their dementia journey, I continue to learn additional care techniques. To bring the new techniques to readers of this edition, I created "The Dementia-Aware Guide to Caregiving," which appears at the end of the book (after chapter 19). Here you will find brief examples of common challenges, followed by different options for providing loving care in that specific scenario. This feature of the book allows you to spend a few moments thinking through how you might respond in these situations. You may decide to change just one or two things in your caregiving approach—and that may make a big difference right away for you, your loved one, and your relationship.

When you become a caregiver for someone with dementia, whatever its cause, the key is to shift your mindset to becoming more dementia-aware. Doing so will help you to transform your dementia care experience from crisis to comfort. After each opportunity to raise awareness and understanding about how dementia impacts individuals, their families, and their communities, I have been gratified to witness enhanced feelings of hope and comfort for all involved.

My experience, observations, and research over years of working with family and professional caregivers, as well as dementia-challenged adults, have shown me that using the affirmative response method of communication, in combination with the stress-management tools and the fresh dementia-aware insights described in this book, help caregivers experience many more meaningful moments with the person they are caring for. I believe that you *can* allow yourself to experience a lasting sense of relief, and that communication and stress management are the crucial ingredients in doing so. I work with family and professional caregivers as a consultant, often assisting with difficult behaviors and developing a care plan. Whenever I use a tried-and-true technique from my program and have a successful outcome, the observing caregiver will ask me something like: "How did you do that? Mom doesn't respond to me that way." I immediately explain that I am able to enter the situation from an outside perspective, without the limitations of the baggage that develops over many years of a long relationship. My perspective allows me to view more than just the single dimension of the "elephant" that is immediately obvious: the dementia and the undesired behavior. Unlike a frustrated, on-the-verge-of-burning-out caregiver who may project negativity, I am able to come in with a fresh approach, and the person with dementia is more receptive.

This does not mean that only someone from outside of the relationship can achieve the same results. Regardless of the current dynamic between you and your loved one or client, you can enjoy positive results by approaching the situation from a new angle. Repeatedly I have seen the benefits of viewing the "elephant" from a broader perspective while still keeping key principles in mind. The case studies you are about to read will help you develop a new perspective. As you apply the techniques in this book, celebrate even the smallest accomplishments and moments of heartfelt connection.

I wish it were possible for me to spend time with all of my readers and to learn from you. It is my hope that through this book I will enter your home or your professional caregiving setting and work alongside you. You will find valuable information from my own experiences and from those of the hundreds of caregivers with whom I have had the honor of working.

To complement this book, I highly recommend that all caregivers connect with additional resources. The Lone Ranger made quite a name for himself, but caregiving should never be a solo role. Reach out to your community and ask for help from professional care providers, gerontologists, social workers, educators, physicians, nurses, nationwide organizations such as the Alzheimer's Association, senior centers, caregiver resource centers, caregiver support group facilitators, family members, neighbors, and other caregivers who are in similar situations. Every day, special people in these positions teach me something new and helpful.

As you read about the affirming responses practiced by countless lay caregivers and professional care providers, you will, I hope, grant yourself a creative license to develop your own personal care plan—to create resourceful and imaginative methods to provide better care for your loved one or client, and for yourself.

We are now embarking on this journey together, and we will meet many amazing and inspiring people along the way.

CHAPTER TWO

Peggy

The Ultimate Toll

🍃 🍃 🍃

With Alicia Murray

Peggy was a wonderful mother of five, grandmother of fourteen, and wife to her husband, Jack. Over the years, Peggy and Jack had carefully planned for a fun retirement. Their goal was to spend time with the kids and grandkids and travel all over the United States. They had decided years before that they would sell their home at retirement, buy a recreational vehicle, and live the carefree life. And that's what they did, visiting their relatives scattered all over the West and square dancing everywhere they went. After fifteen years in the RV, Peggy sensed that the change to a larger, more stable home was on the horizon. Her large and growing family could not stay with her in the RV, and she needed more space to entertain them.

Also, Jack's health and eyesight had started to decline, and Peggy had to do more of the driving. So Peggy and Jack made the decision to sell their home on wheels. They found a double-wide mobile home in a small town in northeastern Colorado, which they could afford on their limited budget. It had the disadvantage of being located far away from the hospitals, doctors, and senior services, but it had the advantage of being next door to their best friends of forty years. They happily settled in.

Three years passed and Peggy started to have conversations with her children about Jack's memory loss and other symptoms of dementia. Some of her friends had been caregivers of spouses with dementia, and she had seen what a hard and stressful job it was. Her daughter offered to help, but Peggy insisted she was okay and would alert her if his condition became unmanageable.

Two weeks after this conversation, disaster struck. When Jack and Peggy sat down to dinner, Peggy suffered a massive heart attack. Jack's reactions to this emergency were slowed by his dementia, which was far more advanced than anyone had realized. By the time the neighbors called 911 and the EMTs arrived from the far-away emergency services, Peggy was already gone.

Lessons Learned

After Peggy's sudden death, the family realized what a high level of care she had been giving Jack twenty-four hours a day, seven days a week, for several years. The common tragedy of sudden caregiver illness or death illustrates why stress management is so important for caregivers. Caring for a person with dementia is described by the National Family Caregivers Association as being three times more work (and stress) than caring for someone with other types of illnesses. It is a long journey, and if caregivers do not take time for themselves, they will not be around to care for the person with dementia.

Peggy's case is a classic example of the devastating effects of caregiver stress. She was not able to paint a precise picture of how much care Jack was receiving (or how much she herself needed) or to ask for help, even though family, neighbors, and friends had continually offered to help over the years. She was just doing what she had always done, believing she could do it alone. It ended up taking her life.

The sheer amount of work caregivers perform can be overwhelming. For the dementia-challenged adult, basic activities of daily living (ADLs) such as bathing, toileting, and dressing become hard to manage. Many caregivers get so involved in helping that they forget how important they are as the caregiver.

In case my message remains unclear, let me say it again: *If you do not take care of yourself, you will not be able to care for your loved one or client!*

When I teach my caregiver training classes, I often ask family caregivers a simple question: "Who is the most important person?" I am frequently amazed to hear silence in the room; caregivers struggle with that question because they always put the dementia-challenged care recipients first. After all, it is their job to take care of their loved ones and clients, not to take care of themselves. Right?

Wrong. Caregivers are often uncomfortable with being aware of how they, themselves, are the key ingredient in the caregiving process! At one of my training sessions on communication and stress management, an attendee brought along his wife. I observed that she was showing early signs of dementia, and during our class I asked that same question, "Who is the most important person?" His wife was the first to answer, as she lovingly pointed to her husband and said, with a smile, "He is!" She knew, even in her dementia, how important her husband was in that caregiver–care recipient relationship. Learn to take care of *you* as well as your loved one. Learn how to manage and cope with stress along the caregiving journey.

Perceptions and Approaches

My years of observations and interactions have taught me that communicating with the dementia-challenged person involves much more than the words coming out of your mouth. Most of the communication comes from tone of voice, facial expression, and body language. Adults with dementia communicate on the basis of emotions.

Many caregivers do not relate the stress that they are feeling to the trying behaviors the dementia-challenged person is exhibiting, when in fact dementia-challenged people are like a mirror of emotions. For example, if you try to rush them with "Hurry up" or "We don't have time," you will experience resistance in the form of slowed responses or a lack of interest in getting ready. If you glare, tap your foot with impatience, approach the person with your arms crossed in front of you, or make frustrated gestures or sounds—such as rolling your eyes or sighing—you are likely to see those signals "mirrored" back at you in behaviors.

If you are stressed, anxious, and fatigued, the person with dementia will sense it but will not be able to understand what is causing your emotions. When you can reduce the stress in your life and begin to exist in a place of serenity, you will see the entire caregiving experience begin to transform. This is another reason why it is so important to keep you, the caregiver, in a place of calmness. It is not only for your own benefit (physically and emotionally) but also to help the person for whom you are caring feel safe, secure, and cooperative throughout the caregiving day.

If only I could have reached Peggy before it was too late—but she was my gentle teacher, showing me that selfless caregivers will take on too much, refusing to ask for or accept help. They will try with all their might to keep promises made long ago to their loved ones, such as the marriage promise to love in sickness and in health, even to a point of pushing beyond their own capabilities.

And Peggy's story hits home, right into my own heart. You see, Peggy was my mother and my children's grandmother, our very own family hero. This personal experience has driven my passion for educating all caregivers, both family and professional, in the awareness of caring for themselves, along with providing tips and tools to assist them in effectively caring for memory-challenged adults. My vision is to bring light into the darkness of dementia through support, encouragement, and hope.

CHAPTER THREE

Deborah

A Daughter's Journey

The signs were subtle and appeared only occasionally at first. The devious brain-destroying disease called Alzheimer's crept up unannounced and began stealing my mom a piece at a time. Alzheimer's is a shrewd and cunning enemy, sneaking in and not clearly identifying itself or even declaring a conventional plan of destruction. "Maybe she's just getting old," I told myself when I first started seeing the symptoms. This was my first bout of dementia-denial, convincing myself it was all a passing nuisance and "no big deal." Then, over time, the progressive failing of her abilities, contrasting from what had been typical for her, began to be more visible. Mom started having more and more difficulty keeping up with mealtime conversations, or she would get easily distracted when performing everyday tasks like cleaning up after a dinner, uncharacteristically leaving dirty dishes on the table or forgetting to put away leftovers. Yet I still found ways to deny the possibility that this was dementia. After all, she still had a pretty good memory.

While she was exhibiting some occasional short-term memory loss, she could still recall crystal-clear details from her past. And she was often willing and able to perform detailed familiar tasks to completion or engage in conversation like usual. Just when I would feel a sense of ease, I would witness her struggle to recall the right words when talking about an article she had just read in the newspaper or faltering with the fine points and details when she was discussing a thought or idea. In the beginning, Mom would compensate by changing the subject or replacing the elusive thought or word with another. And when I would observe her compensating, I would tell myself she was experiencing an occasional brain interruption—we all have those, right? But then she started having a problem understanding and following even a simple plot or storyline on a television show. Still fueled by denial, my inner voice would say, "She is just tired," or, "Perhaps she is having trouble hearing the television—it was her hearing, right?" Back and forth I volleyed my feelings of acceptance that this was short lived and would be "fixed" by waiting it out. But I was plagued by fear that even more indisputable failings would rear their ugly heads. I would search for solace by convincing myself that my feelings of denial were justified whenever Mom would have her "moments of clarity" and appear to me as her "normal self."

I want to pause for a moment and make it clear that I did not have a sudden profound moment of acceptance that this situation was serious and getting worse. My lack of "dementia-awareness" kept me in this roller coaster state of perplexity for a very long time. It did not help that Mom's slow decline was spread out over several years, and this lengthy span slowed my own cognizance that this situation went far beyond just "getting old." Her gradual decline kept "fooling me" until the symptoms became unmistakable. Yes, even though I saw my mom struggling to maintain her very being and saw her clearly overwhelmed with even familiar and everyday tasks, I still sought out the emotional safety of my illusory place within denial. About a year into this journey, I had insisted that Mom see her doctor about these early symptoms. I went with her to this initial appointment, and we both received his toned-down diagnosis of "mild cognitive impairment." When we did not hear the dreaded word "Alzheimer's," the news was perceived by both of us as not so bad—certainly no need to panic or worry. After all, "mild cognitive impairment" is not as serious as "Alzheimer's" or "dementia," right?

This "benign" diagnosis also did not push me to be aware of the need to know more in order to make good care decisions from the beginning. I wanted to believe that I could fix her, or change the progression, or stop the decline. I wanted to believe it would go away, she would get better, and that I would not have to go toe to toe with this relentless monster. I continued to lean on the defense mechanism of denial, justifying my feelings again and again whenever Mom would tap into her diminishing cognitive abilities and misstep, or when she would access the portion of her presently unscathed brain function and appear normal. It was in these "normal" moments that I would feel validated that her symptoms were really not that bad, just "mild cognitive impairment" and not the scary "D" word, dementia, at all.

But what was really happening was that I was moving in and out of acceptance and self-deception. So I just kept "observing," "taking note," and turning my head, attempting to fix it all in my mind. I continued to implement inadequate short-term solutions such as using sticky notes or verbal reminders, and even correcting Mom when she did not get a detail or word right, forgot to take her medication, or did not remember something I had just told her.

Of course, gradually the cruel progression of the dementia took over, and no sticky notes or verbal reminders or corrections or short in-and-out visits could withstand the dementia's devastating impact on her mind. Mom would get very anxious when I would show up at her door, even though I had told her an hour before I was on my way. She would mix up her medications, taking them at the wrong time or not at all. She even stopped taking a shower and changing her clothes regularly. Visit after visit I observed her wearing the same dirty black turtleneck, black sweatpants, and gloves (even inside the house, as she was always complaining of the cold, even in the heat of summer). She also was having more physical difficulties—losing her balance, shuffling and falling often. I would notice bruises and injuries, and when I would ask her about them, she could not explain where they had come from or remember where or when or if she had fallen.

Then late one night I got a call from a neighbor. They had found Mom wandering out in her driveway in her nightgown, obviously in a state of extreme confusion. It was suddenly undeniably clear that she could not be left alone, so I resolved to move in with her.

After that difficult life-changing decision, it became almost impossible to find consolation in ignoring the inevitable or turning the other way. My unrealistic rationalizations—based in desperate denial—could no longer hide the horrible reality that this was dementia—progressive and permanent loss of her vital brain functions. Mom's increasing loss of ability made me sit up and take notice full time now. Yet my new-found awareness only unearthed the fact that it was also challenging and expensive to find help. I soon discovered that no one had yet developed a simple test for Alzheimer's or for most of the other 100+ causes of dementia. Although there was ongoing research and new technology allowing for more detailed brain imaging, these tests still only gave clues and allowed for better educated guesses about the causes of brain function loss. Mom's primary doctor did not feel comfortable diagnosing the cause as Alzheimer's disease or another possible cause of her dementia symptoms without enough evidence from more comprehensive testing, so we were referred to a neurologist who specialized in dementia. In my quest to become more "dementia-aware," I learned that there is no one simple test to tell you if your loved one has it or not. Though medical professionals could gather clues from symptoms and draw reasonable conclusions from them, there was no easy, precise, or clear-cut path to a diagnosis.

When Mom's symptoms became so challenging she could no longer manage her memory loss without constant supervision and care, then and only then did I accept the true and realistic fact that she had permanent and progressive loss of normal brain function—in other words, dementia! This is when I came out from under the umbrella of denial and knew what really counted. It did not matter so much about what the diagnosis was or the cause of her growing list of dementia symptoms; it mattered more to me how well she could function and how my role was now one of dealing directly with what I saw, taking action, and developing an effective care plan. It was crucial that this plan be grounded in care strategies such as: staying in the moment with her; providing her with appropriate emotional, personal, and physical care; keeping her safe; and managing her complicated symptoms and behaviors.

I now look back and realize that had I been "dementia-aware" from the beginning, I could have saved myself and, more importantly, my mom, much aggravation and anxiety on this journey. How I wish I had known then what I have learned since.

Lessons Learned

It is human to deny what we find unpleasant or frightening. But when denial prevents us from seeing facts and facing their implications, it will not help us or our loved ones. In most countries, there is a lack of awareness and understanding of dementia, resulting in stigma and barriers to diagnosis and care, both of which negatively impact caregivers, families, and societies—physically, psychologically, and economically. Dementia is overwhelming not only for the people who have it, but also for their caregivers, family members, and local communities.

Because nobody wants a loved one to have dementia, caregivers are vulnerable to a particular kind of denial. I call it "dementia-denial," and it is based in both self-defense and self-protection. Ultimately, denial will make the dementia care journey much more treacherous. Dementia-denial causes a caregiver to go along with the person's insistence that he or she is "fine" or "normal." Caregivers in dementia-denial often continue to let loved ones make risky decisions, such as driving a car or overseeing finances far longer than is safe, and neglect to develop a legal and financial plan to step in as the decision-maker. Dementia-denial is a hindrance to putting systems in place to protect against many kinds of potentially dangerous abnormal behaviors, allowing them to continue unchecked until someone is injured.

The antidote for "dementia-denial" is to become "dementia-aware." A caregiver who is dementia-aware is one who understands that he or she must seek education about his or her loved one's condition. A dementia-aware caregiver displays a high level of knowledge of the many moving parts of dementia symptoms, the multitude of causes, and tools to adapt and respond. A dementia-aware caregiver gets help in order to make sure that he or she will have sustained energy and resilience during the dementia-care marathon. Choosing to operate from a place of acceptance instead of denial is a vital part of being a dementia-aware caregiver.

Perceptions and Approaches

Here's what becoming a dementia-aware caregiver looks like:

• *Dementia-aware caregivers access support from the medical community.* Denying that there are dementia symptoms can delay getting treatment and an appropriate care plan for an individual. Such delays in treatment may allow dangerous declines in health and well-being. This can make dementia more difficult to treat and have consequences on overall quality of life—for both the person with dementia and you, the caregiver. If initial testing only results in a diagnosis of "early dementia" or "mild cognitive impairment," it is not a signal to the caregiver and other family members that everything is okay and no one needs to plan ahead. This is still a serious situation that may and probably will get worse. Neurologists and primary care physicians experienced in dementia need ample time to run tests and assess each individual patient's symptoms. And most of the medications to help with dementia symptoms work best if they are given when the symptoms are exhibited and monitored early on in the dementia journey.

• *Dementia-aware caregivers remain open to continuing education about their loved ones' conditions.* You may have learned a lot about dementia initially, but it is important to stay ahead of the curve and keep learning, as a progressive dementia will continue to alter and diminish your loved one's abilities. Most forms of dementia are progressive, which means every month/day/moment can bring changes. The hard reality is that the definition of "normal" must be continually revised. The higher your level of knowledge early on in the care journey, the more accepting and aware you will be as a caregiver. Maintain realistic expectations that these changes will happen so you can remain fluid and flexible in your care plan and approach.

• *Dementia-aware caregivers consider the bigger picture.* It is not just about your loved one's life. Consider the safety of your loved one and others who might be affected, such as other drivers or pedestrians on the road. While we understand that losing a driver's license is a particularly uncomfortable situation for most people to talk about, it is important to understand that denial has a ripple effect on others.

• *Dementia-aware caregivers continuously reach out to stay supported all along the way.* It is important to be sustained by family, neighbors, friends, and other caregivers through support groups, professionals in the community, and ongoing education. *It takes a village to care for a loved one with dementia.* Once dementia-denial has been alleviated by dementia-awareness, family members and professionals can begin to seek the best avenues available for treatment and care for their loved ones, clients, or residents with dementia.

Dementia-awareness must go well beyond the individual family or professional caregiver, even to those who are not presently on a personal dementia care journey. Millions of Americans are already affected by this disease, and that number is expected to rapidly grow during the coming decades. As a society, we must become more dementia-aware and able to direct caregivers and persons with dementia to appropriate support resources. And that starts by being dementia-aware on an individual level.

Denial from the viewpoint of a caregiver is an entirely different experience than denial from the perspective of the person who has dementia. In the next chapter, Charles's story provides insight into why the person with dementia is also often challenged by denial and how you can navigate this dynamic as a caregiver.

CHAPTER FOUR

Charles

There Is Nothing Wrong with Me

My father, Charles, is a perfect case study and example of the initial acceptance of a dementia diagnosis followed by the relentless change to an apparent dementia-denial of the disease as it progressed.

Charles himself initiated the visit to his primary care physician that resulted in his diagnosis. On his own, he had become increasingly aware of the insidious dementia signs and symptoms before I had even noticed them. At the doctor's appointment, my father was able to discuss with his physician how he was experiencing some sleep difficulties, slowed movements and slight tremors, as well as decline in his cognitive function and ability to process information that had always come so easily to him in the past. Sadly, it turned out to be early-stage Lewy Body dementia. At that time he accepted the doctor's verdict with poise. My father and I talked about it, researched it, and made plans together about what we would do. We decided to make the most of the time we had left before the disease started taking over his mind and abilities. By making accommodations for the short-term memory loss and other budding symptoms, we managed to enjoy a few years spending precious time and making special memories—doing all those things we had put off before we received the dreadful diagnosis.

The progression was mercifully slow but painfully steady, especially at the beginning. But over time, the disease began to assume control of his life. His personality changed entirely. If I even brought up the idea of visiting a doctor for any reason, he would become furious. I did not understand what was happening, why my father was changing before my eyes. I had to accept the heart-wrenching reality that this was no longer the father I once knew. The ever-present smile and loving disposition was all but completely gone. The gentle, patient man who for fifty-six years had never had an ill-tempered word for me now frequently exploded with irrational angry outbursts and uncharacteristic fits of impatience.

It was in the final part of his dementia journey that he became completely unaware of how debilitated he had become. He could no longer remember or process that he had been given the diagnosis early on, or that at one time he had even gracefully accepted the fact. At this point, he had full-blown dementia-denial of his own illness. But this went beyond the normal type of denial so many people experience when facing difficult circumstances, such as the denial I had as a caregiver. Instead, my father had a different kind of denial known as *anosognosia*— literally a lack of knowledge of disease. I later learned that anosognosia [an-o'so-no'zhah] has long been recognized in people with strokes, brain tumors, Alzheimer's, Lewy Body, and Huntington's disease, as well as many of the other causes of dementia symptoms. Although this dementia-denial may at first appear to be similar to the denial the caregiver is experiencing, anosognosia is not the same and is far more challenging. Unfortunately, there is no antidote for anosognosia, as there is no way to challenge it with dementia-awareness.

As his son, I was forced to watch my father fade away a piece at a time without having any way to stop it, change it, fix it, or console him by sharing what was happening. Any mention of dementia, Lewy Body, the decline in his health and abilities, or his progressing care needs would send my father into a rage: "There is nothing wrong with me!" His resistance to my care efforts was nothing short of intense, often with a pinch of paranoia and a handful of spitefulness thrown into the mix. Any attempt on my part to make him understand that he had changed and needed to accept new limits was an exercise in frustration for both of us. It was simply much more successful if as his primary caregiver I made all decisions related to his care without discussing them with him or asking for his input or opinion.

On a very basic level, I came to realize my father's "thinker" was broken and that the more I did the "thinking" for him, the kinder and more supportive I remained in his eyes. This all felt weird and crazy, and so contrary to how I had identified my part in this father-son relationship, yet I found that when I changed my communication approach and shared less information concerning his condition and necessary care decisions, he appeared calmer and more at peace. When I finally recognized that he simply "did not know what he did not know" and I accepted that I must do all the "knowing" for him about his care, our dementia journey became less tumultuous, and we were able to experience many more meaningful moments together.

Lessons Learned

In some cases, people with dementia will experience precisely the same kind of dementia-denial their caregivers exhibit, namely that understandable emotional desire to convince ourselves that everything is fine. However, anosognosia is an entirely different problem. While anosognosia is still difficult to define, researchers know it results from physical, anatomical changes or damage to the part of the brain that affects perception of one's own illness. As a neurological impairment, it is common following brain injuries or diseases. For instance, people with a disease or illness causing dementia may display anosognosia and insist they do not have a problem. Naturally, the family member or professional caregiver who has to deal with this problem can become exasperated.

To make the situation even more challenging, anosognosia may be complete or selective, in the latter case only revealing itself in certain situations that trigger the person's dementia-denial, such as when he or she becomes frustrated trying to perform simple daily tasks. The person diagnosed with any form of dementia may be entirely unaware of his or her impairment, or react with anger and defensiveness if confronted about the illness. This makes it difficult to diagnose anosognosia and tough to differentiate it from common dementia-denial. But whether your loved one is in simple denial of his or her dementia or has anosognosia, the most effective caregiving strategy is one of acceptance and empathy toward the symptoms and subsequent behaviors, rather than endlessly trying (and failing) to make the person with dementia understand.

Much more than denial, anosognosia is a far-reaching lack of awareness of impairment—most people do not even know they are ill—and it affects up to 81 percent of people with Alzheimer's disease, the leading cause of dementia. After strokes, some studies show up to 77 percent of people suffer anosognosia. And just like any and all causes and symptoms of dementia, this lack of awareness affects each person differently.

Anosognosia with dementia shows no favoritism with regard to occupation, gender, ethnicity, education, or financial status, as evidenced in the life of President Woodrow Wilson and his personal dementia journey. In 1919, toward the end of his second term, President Wilson suffered a stroke. Following his stroke, the notable feature of the President's behavior was his denial of his incapacity. Denial of illness is a common sequel to the type of brain injury received by President Wilson. In this condition, the patient denies or appears unaware of such physical deficits as paralysis or blindness, as well as loss of other brain functions. To casual observers, anosognosic patients may appear normal and even bright and witty. When not talking about their disability, they can be quite rational, and tests of their intelligence may show no deficit. In President Wilson's case, his anosognosia prevented him from getting the care he needed after his stroke.

Wilson described himself as "lame" and referred to his cane as his "third leg," but otherwise he considered himself perfectly fit to be president. There was even talk of a third term. Yet his close associates noticed a change in his personality and abilities. He became increasingly suspicious, even paranoid, without having the dimmest awareness of the fact that he was perhaps becoming a different person from who he once was. Stockton Axson, his brother-in-law from his first marriage, wrote that President Wilson "would be seized with what, to a normal person, would seem to be inexplicable outbursts of emotion. He was furious at anyone who suggested that he had physical and mental problems, and the last months of his presidency became a graveyard of fired associates."

To explain this type of dementia-denial another way, "Our right brain is wired to detect anomalies and new information and incorporate these into our sense of reality," according to neuroscientist Dr. V. S. Ramachandran, in the *New York Times*. When something happens to damage that part of the brain—such as a stroke, Alzheimer's, or many of the other causes of dementia—then "the left brain seeks to maintain continuity of belief, using denial, rationalization, confabulation and other tricks to keep one's mental model of the world intact."

If you are concerned that your loved one, client, or resident might have dementia complicated by anosognosia, here are some signs to look for:

- Not keeping up with regular daily tasks or personal hygiene.
- Having difficulty managing money or bills.
- Being more spontaneous or less inhibited in conversation without concern for his or her own behavior.
- Becoming angry when confronted with forgetfulness, lack of self-care, poor decision-making, or many other dementia symptoms.
- Confabulating: making up answers that the person believes are true, though sometimes the details may be imaginary, may pertain to something that happened in the past, or even be based on something he or she read or heard elsewhere.

Perceptions and Approaches

Dealing with dementia-denial on the part of the person with dementia is a trying situation for caregivers, who are endeavoring to help someone who essentially does not and cannot acknowledge he or she is ill. People with dementia and anosognosia exhibit obvious difficulties with routine tasks, judgment, and executive thinking skills, yet they often insist they do not need help, even to the point of refusing medical evaluation or treatment, as well as much-needed non-medical assistance and emotional support.

For caregivers, successfully overcoming dementia-denial involves the ability to learn a new perception and deeper understanding of dementia, and then take that knowledge to develop a care approach that works. People with dementia and anosognosia, however, cannot become dementia-aware, as they will become progressively more incapable of recognizing they have any dementia symptoms, even when their symptoms are very obvious to those who are caring for them. Unlike with caregiver dementia-denial, there is no remedy for the form of denial exhibited by someone with anosognosia.

It is a scary thought to consider. What if you were ill, suffering from dementia, and did not know it? And there was no way to make you understand the complexity of it all? How would your loved ones or treatment providers give you appropriate care if you continued to refuse their well-intentioned and necessary help? This is precisely what many caregivers experience as the person whom they are assisting continues to resist critical support on many different levels. This often leaves the caregiver with the responsibility of providing and accessing appropriate help—having to make difficult decisions without the buy-in from the one who desperately needs increasing levels of care.

For example, many anguished family caregivers have contacted me about how and when to take away the car keys, while their loved one with dementia is still certain he or she can safely operate an automobile. Another common question concerns when it is time to access out-of-home care. People with dementia and anosognosia will dig in their heels and wholly believe they can stay independent in their own homes and safely care for themselves, even when all the evidence strongly suggests otherwise. Answering these questions and determining the "right time" can be excruciating for the primary caregiver and is another reason why dementia care is such a stressful role. In these situations, you, the caregiver, must cease basing essential care decisions upon what you believe your loved one wants—instead, you must move to the logical response of decisions based on what he or she needs at the time, accessing the care and assistance that will keep your loved one, and everyone around your loved one, safe. Going against your loved one's wishes is seldom the path of least resistance—

on the contrary, it is almost always the path of greatest opposition. And it is an exhausting uphill segment of the dementia journey. But if your loved one has both dementia and dementia-denial—especially denial in the form of anosognosia—it is essential that you take charge of his or her affairs.

Here are five things to keep in mind when caring for someone with dementia symptoms and anosognosia:

1. *Use positive action statements in your communication.* Be gentle, encouraging, and empathetic about necessary tasks. Avoid asking too many questions or giving too many options. Questions can be distressing at the best of times and can put pressure on people. Questions, reasoning, and multiple options become too much information for the person with dementia to process. KEEP IT SIMPLE!

2. *Spend time with no pressure, no agenda, no judgment, and no expectations.* Allow the person to be whoever he or she is right now. Downsize any responsibilities that are unnecessary. Often the answer is a professional in-home caregiver, adult day care, or a memory care community that is trained in dementia care. It takes a village to care for someone with dementia, so build your village of care professionals, family, friends, and local community members. Remember, you cannot stop, change, or cure the dementia symptoms—you can only help to manage them.

3. *Avoid fact- and reason-based discussions with the person who has dementia symptoms and anosognosia* about his or her medical condition or changing care needs. The more you, the caregiver, become dementia-aware, the more you will see that your loved one's comments, behaviors, and changes are an expected part of the disease process and out of his or her control, helping you to better plan and accept what is yet to come. When voicing concerns, stay calm, confident, patient, and present in the moment. Articulate your thoughts in a simple and positive light. Practice communication that excludes discussion about what abilities he or she has lost, all the while increasing the focus and attention on what abilities still remain.

4. *Allow people with dementia the dignity of experiencing whatever emotions they are feeling at the time,* with an understanding that these

feelings are real to them, even if they are difficult for you to understand. Although people with dementia may seem distant or confused at times, their emotions and feelings remain. When interacting with people who have dementia, hold their hands, give them a hug. Show them patience, compassion, and care. Attempting to correct or reason with a person who has anosognosia will only result in resistance—a test of frustration for both of you that can generate further feelings of anxiety, even accelerating to more extreme challenging behaviors, such as combativeness and aggression.

5. *Be sure you remember to take care of yourself.* Caregivers often feel obligated to sacrifice themselves for the sake of the person for whom they are caring. As a result of neglecting to care for themselves, caregivers frequently become burned out and resentful, especially if other family members do not share the burden. Holding regular family meetings and keeping open communication can help clear the air before things reach a breaking point. It is essential to everyone's well-being that you remain in good health and can balance your care responsibilities with your own needs.

As you continue to read this book, you will become more and more dementia-aware, helping to sustain you through the many obstacles you will encounter on the road ahead. Whether you are a family caregiver, a professional caregiver, or an individual who wishes to help build a more dementia-aware world, keep in mind that the more you know about the many layers of dementia, the better you will be able not only to navigate your own dementia care journey, but to help others on their personal journeys as well.

CHAPTER FIVE

Frances

What Is Dementia?

Frances walked by with short, scuffling steps. Her body was stooped over; she looked down, not ahead. She seemed unaware of me as she passed, just inches away. She wore a distant look on her weather-worn face and a blank stare in her glazed eyes, but I knew she was aware of my presence. So I said her name.

She paused, lifted her head, and answered, "Yes?" I asked, "Frances, does it feel like you are dreaming?" Suddenly aware and alert, she looked me in the eye and said, "Absolutely!" Then she slowly turned, her eyes and face as empty as before, and shuffled away.

I had spent several hours with Frances over the previous few weeks and had become aware that she often looked like a sleepwalker, not thoroughly in the same awake existence as I was, but still able to converse or relate to me in my reality for spurts of time. Frances was in the advanced stages of Alzheimer's disease and was being assisted lovingly by her only son, who had quit his job to care for her full time.

Her son had contacted me to help him manage some of her challenging behaviors, including her repetitive daily routine and her restlessness during the late evening into nighttime, a phenomenon commonly called sundowning.

Frances slept only two to three hours at night, and during the day she was agitated and restless. She busied herself by taking all of the cups, bowls, and glasses out of the kitchen cabinets, filling them with warm water, and then placing them on the counters, table, and even on the floor. She would then involve herself with her other routine of taking everything out of her closet, spreading clothes and shoes on her bed and on the floor, often taking everything off the hangers and making piles. She never sat down. To get her to eat, her son placed finger foods on a plate on the corner of the table, since she would only eat on the go.

I was curious about Frances's profession before her retirement, and I was fascinated to learn that she had been a baker. For the majority of her life, her daily routine had begun long before sunrise when she would start the yeast processing in warm water. In addition to working as a baker, she had managed a large acreage property. Her son told me about his fond memories of her quick, long strides as she gardened, mowed, picked, and watered to keep her treasured land in tip-top shape.

She had always been busy, busy, busy—driven by her parents' sayings, such as "The devil finds work for idle hands!" My initial observation was that although the son was coping with her care, he was showing many signs of extreme stress. He was exhausted from the constant interruptions at night and lack of sleep.

My first suggestion was for him to seek out and use regular in-home care and respite. He needed to take time to rest and sleep without his mom continually interrupting him. He also needed time for himself, away from his caregiving responsibilities, to do things he enjoyed. And because knowledge is empowering, he needed to carve out time to get specialized information about dementia and learn more about his mom's illness. With a better understanding of dementia and the behaviors it may cause, the son could customize Frances's care to take into account her distinctive history and needs.

⤜᷅⤛

Lessons Learned

The word *dementia* comes from the Latin *dis*, meaning "away from," and *mens*, meaning "mind." It describes a state of being away from your mind or existing in this world while being away from your previous life. Like sleepwalking.

Dementia in its various manifestations (for example, issues with cognition, behavior, mood, psychological state, muscle memory, etc.) is a *symptom*, very much like a cough or a fever is a symptom of the flu. If you have a cough, it does not necessarily mean you have lung cancer, and if you have dementia, it does not necessarily mean the cause of your dementia symptoms is Alzheimer's disease. The cough could be a symptom of respiratory influenza, and dementia could be one of several symptoms caused by a stroke, for example. Dementia is often confused with Alzheimer's. But Alzheimer's is a disease (a cause), and the various manifestations of dementia are symptoms, either of the leading cause of dementia—Alzheimer's disease—or of another disease or disorder or even exposure to a toxin. If you had a medical exam and the doctor gave you the dreaded news that you were suffering from dementia, the next question you would need to ask is, "What is causing this dementia?"

As explained by the Alzheimer's Association, "dementia is not a specific disease. It's an overall term that describes a wide range of symptoms associated with a decline in memory or other thinking skills severe enough to reduce a person's ability." For example, an exposure to anesthesia increases the risk of dementia, although anesthesia-induced dementia is usually temporary. Chemical or other exposure is often misdiagnosed or overlooked as a cause of dementia. According to ICARA (Investigative Clinical Amyloid Research in Alzheimer's), the medications or substances that may cause dementia include the following:

- alcohol
- amphetamines
- atropine (a drug used in anesthesia)
- barbiturates
- bromides (an ingredient in some medications)
- certain anti-Parkinsonian drugs
- certain antispasmodics
- certain tranquilizers
- manganese poisoning
- cocaine (including "crack" cocaine)

- cortisone
- digitalis
- illicit drugs
- lead poisoning
- lithium
- mercury poisoning

Drug interactions and drug withdrawal can also cause dementia, although it is usually temporary.

In addition, there is a difference between dementia and delirium. Although the symptoms of dementia and delirium are similar, the causes and definitions are not. Dementia is defined as an irreversible state of cognitive impairment and short-term memory loss caused by organic brain disease—most commonly Alzheimer's disease or multiple cerebral infarcts (strokes). Delirium, on the other hand, is a state of cognitive impairment, clouding of consciousness, and confusion that improves when the cause is addressed.

Delirium is characterized by a sudden onset of confusion. Symptoms of delirium occur rapidly—not over a long period of time, as happens with dementia. According to the *Merck Manual for Healthcare Professionals*, the most common causes of delirium are

- certain medications—particularly anticholinergics, psycho-active drugs, and opioids
- dehydration
- infection (such as urinary tract infection)

There are some circumstances that can cause people to develop dementia-like symptoms. Depression, dehydration, malnutrition, hospitalization from a severe injury or fall—all can cause a person to behave abnormally. I advise many caregivers to get a thorough medical workup for their loved ones or clients to rule out these other causes of dementia symptoms or delirium. Unfortunately, in contrast to delirium, dementia is a long-term, generally irreversible condition. The most common cause of dementia is Alzheimer's disease; between 60 and 80 percent of people with dementia have Alzheimer's disease. There are, however, many other causes of dementia, including stroke,

Lewy Body disease, Parkinson's disease, and head trauma. Many people have a dual diagnosis, with two or more causes, such as Parkinson's and Alzheimer's, or a stroke and Alzheimer's.

People with dementia may have any of these problems and other problems, as well:

- confusion
- disorientation
- repetitive behaviors
- problems with tracking or processing information
- spatial difficulties, such as having a limited view of physical surroundings
- anxiety
- fear
- paranoia

Nearly everyone with dementia has progressive short-term memory loss. The dementia-challenged person may shuffle and be slightly off balance or have problems with depth perception.

Dementia frequently brings about impaired judgment and a loss of inhibitions, causing individuals to exhibit behaviors that may appear odd and may be out of character for them. In addition, people with dementia may have difficulty making decisions. The person's ability to be organized and to do multiple tasks simultaneously may become limited. Many people with dementia choose not to participate in their usual activities if there are too many outside stimuli.

Do any of these behaviors and problems sound familiar to you as you think about your loved one?

Perceptions and Approaches

As a helpful visualization for understanding the progressive loss of normal brain function, imagine that a healthy human brain is like a block of solid sharp cheddar cheese. In contrast, the brain of a person with dementia looks like a large, traditional wedge of Swiss cheese, with holes spread throughout it. And in the center of that sizeable wedge of perforated Swiss cheese is a hungry rat. The rat in the cheese is the root cause—or source—of the progressive and permanent loss of normal brain function resulting in the growing list of dementia symptoms. In this example, we will name (or diagnose) this rat as Mr. Alzheimer's (a.k.a., the progressive cause of the loss of normal brain function presented as many possible dementia symptoms). Mr. Alzheimer's, in this example, comes in the form of Alzheimer's disease—the leading cause of dementia—yet could come in any of the more than one hundred causes of dementia, such as Parkinson's disease, Lewy Body disease, Huntington's disease, AIDS, or alcoholism. Regardless, the rat is busily eating away at the block of priceless "cheese" (memory, cognitive function, and personality).

At this time, we do not know how Mr. Alzheimer's (or most of the other one hundred causes of loss of normal brain function) initially makes his home in the brain. Unfortunately, we also do not have any way to get the rat out, or halt or even slow the damage he causes. And the rat continues running around to all different sections of the brain, nibbling away at the cheese and leaving ever larger holes. Mr. Alzheimer's path of destruction is up to his unique discretion—he may choose to steadily move about and then show bursts of energy and quickly change his course, exposing faster and more abrupt declines in the person's abilities. Or the rat may mosey about, instigating a long and mysterious path of deterioration over many months and years. When working with clients and families, I refer to this phenomenon as the "cheese and holes." Sometimes you may enjoy a day of clarity with your loved one, when he or she is "all there"—that is when you have hit the cheese. And on another day, your loved one may be confused, agitated, or even vacant—you have hit a hole in the cheese.

Being a dementia-aware caregiver involves accepting the unfortunate fact that when the effects of permanent, progressive loss of normal brain function are readily observable, there is no way to stop, alter, or fix the escalating dementia symptoms. Instead, the caregiver needs to implement a realistic care approach, with the understanding that you can only do your best to manage the changes. It is critical for a dementia-aware caregiver to stay fluid and flexible, as the strategies for managing the symptoms will shift in the blink of an eye—or in the next greedy bite of cheese.

I want to help you develop the ability to take hold of and cherish every possible connection with the "cheese" that remains—for as long as you can.

Easier said than done, considering the difficulties of caregiving. Your day must be filled with patience, empathy, and efforts to maintain your loved one's dignity. At the same time, you must manage all the day-to-day activities necessary to feed, clothe, bathe, and nurture the person in your care.

Frances was suffering from the short-term memory loss typical of dementia. Along with the memory loss, Frances may also have been experiencing Capgras syndrome. A person with Capgras syndrome, also known as Capgras delusion, believes that people close to her have been replaced by duplicates. The person with Capgras may doubt her own identity and question whether she, in whole or in part, has been replaced by an impostor. This syndrome is more prevalent in women than in men.

Although the syndrome is most common among people with schizophrenia, it can also occur as a result of a severe brain injury or dementia. Its effects may be acute, chronic, or transient. The delusions center around one of the senses—most often sight—and remain localized to that one sense. For example, a man afflicted with Capgras may recognize his wife's voice on the phone yet believe that she is an impostor when he sees her in person.

Whatever the cause in Frances's case, she no longer recognized her son. She confused him with his father (her husband), who had passed away six years earlier. She could no longer process the recollection of her son the way she had before dementia damaged her short-term memories. The son had tried to bring his mom into his reality by explaining that he was her son, but his mother met his efforts with anger and anxiety. He told me that his mother would respond more positively and be more cooperative if he just "went along with her perception and did not argue with her about his identity." He had come to realize through trial and error that he could not win this dispute.

Letting go of the need to try to convince his mother of his identity had paradoxically given him a greater feeling of empowerment.

We all forget things occasionally, but the short-term memory loss caused by dementia is different. The following paragraphs describe how our brains usually store short-term and long-term memories, and how dementia affects our normal memory storage processes.

Imagine a short-term-memory file cabinet appearing every morning on the outer edge of your brain for the memories you will create today—what you ate for breakfast, where you parked your car when you arrived at work, and so on. At the end of the day this cabinet will move in one notch, toward the center of your brain, and be replaced by a new outer-edge file cabinet the next day (and the next, and the next). These more recent files contain the short-term memories. Each file cabinet, as it ages, moves deeper and deeper into the recesses of the brain. As these cabinets age, they become the long-term memories. The ongoing destruction caused by the dementia begins to destroy these files, however, starting with today's file cabinet.

How does it feel to have these recent memories destroyed? Consider this comparison. Almost all of us have gone to the mall, parked, shopped, and returned to the lot only to realize we cannot remember where we left the car. You know how uncomfortable it feels when you can't find your car? You may even start to wonder if it has been stolen. Well, that unpleasant blank feeling and memory deficit is what the dementia-challenged adult feels every day, every hour, every minute. Can you imagine how frightening and disorienting this must be?

If we continue to visualize the rows of memory storage files in the "memory room" of our brains, with the most recent memories in front and the long-ago memories farther and farther back, we can begin to understand how dementia-challenged people lose the ability to access the most recent memories. The fluid (short-term) memory file cabinets disappear, one by one.

Yet people with dementia often maintain the ability to access memories from long ago (known as "crystal memories"), because many of those far-back memory storage files have not yet been deleted by the dementia. Many family caregivers have told me that their family members with dementia can clearly remember detailed events from long ago but cannot remember things that happened yesterday. This is a common experience. It is as if people with dementia are on "rewind" in their memories, like a biographical movie running backwards. Short-term memories start to disappear, while long-ago memories become clearer and may feel like "now," making it easier to confuse twenty-year-old or thirty-year-old memories with the present time.

Understanding how memories are stored and lost makes it easier to understand the memory loss of dementia and how it affects people with dementia every day. Their world becomes a puzzling mix-up of times, feelings, and visions from their past life randomly woven into the present. The good news is that you can still share meaningful moments with your loved one.

The following information from the Alzheimer's Association provides additional details about dementia.

What Is Dementia?
Information Compiled by Denise Davis, Program Director, Alzheimer's Association, Greater Sacramento Area Office

Memory loss that disrupts everyday life is not a normal part of aging. However, there is no clear line that separates normal changes from the warning signs. Because of this uncertainty about what's causing a problem, if a loved one's abilities seem to be declining, it is a good idea to get a diagnosis from a doctor—and from a doctor who specializes in diagnosing dementia, if possible.

According to the Alzheimer's Association, these are the 10 warning signs of dementia:

1. Memory Loss. This is when a person's immediate memory is being challenged. Forgetting recently learned information is one of the most common signs of dementia.
2. Difficulty Performing Familiar Tasks. People with dementia often find it hard to plan or complete everyday tasks. Individuals may lose track of the steps involved in

preparing a meal, placing a telephone call, or playing a game.

3. Problems with Language. People with Alzheimer's disease may often forget simple words or substitute unusual words, making their speech or writing hard to understand. They may be unable to find the fork, for example, and instead ask for "that thing for my mouth."

4. Disorientation to Time and Place. Persons with Alzheimer's disease can become lost in their own neighborhoods, forget where they are and how they got there, and not know how to get back home.

5. Poor or Decreased Judgment. Those with Alzheimer's may dress inappropriately, wearing several layers on a warm day or little clothing in the cold. They may show poor judgment about money, like giving away large sums to telemarketers.

6. Problems with Abstract Thinking. Someone with Alzheimer's disease may have unusual difficulty performing complex mental tasks; for example, they may forget what numbers are and how they should be used.

7. Misplacing Things. A person with Alzheimer's disease may put things in unusual places—a high-heeled shoe in the freezer or a necklace in the sugar bowl.

8. Changes in Mood or Behavior. Someone with Alzheimer's disease may show rapid mood swings—from calm to tears to anger—for no apparent reason.

9. Changes in Personality. The personalities of people with dementia can change dramatically. They may become extremely confused, suspicious, fearful, or dependent on a family member.

10. Loss of Initiative. A person with Alzheimer's disease may become very passive, sitting in front of the TV for hours, sleeping more than usual, or not wanting to do normal activities.

Dementia is a general term for a group of brain disorders, and Alzheimer's is the most common type of dementia, accounting for 60 to 80 percent of those with dementia.

How can you tell whether someone's symptoms are a sign of normal aging or are a sign of dementia? There are some specific signs. For example, all types of dementia involve mental decline that

- is a step down from a higher level of functioning (for example, the person did not always have a poor memory);
- is severe enough to interfere with usual activities and daily life; and
- affects more than one of the following four core mental abilities:
  - recent memory (the ability to learn and recall new information)
  - language (the ability to write or speak, or to understand written or spoken words)
  - visuospatial function (the brain's ability to translate visual signals into an accurate impression of where objects are located in space, and the ability to understand and use symbols, maps, etc.)
  - executive function (the ability to plan, reason, solve problems, and focus on a task).

There are over seventy types of dementia. Some of the more widely known types are

- Alzheimer's disease
- mild cognitive impairment (MCI), a pre-dementia state
- mixed dementia: Alzheimer's disease and vascular dementia occurring at the same time
- dementia with Lewy bodies (Lewy Body dementia)
- Parkinson's disease
- frontotemporal dementia (Pick's disease)
- Creutzfeldt-Jakob disease (CJD)
- normal pressure hydrocephalus (NPH)
- Huntington's disease (HD)
- Wernicke-Korsakoff syndrome

The various types of dementia have different warning signs, rates of progression, and behaviors, which is one reason it's important to get an accurate diagnosis of the type of dementia. An accurate diagnosis means that the person with dementia and his or her caregivers can learn more about the likely (though not certain) progression in a person with that specific kind of dementia. Medications can help relieve some of the more troubling behaviors for certain kinds of dementia; these medications are especially useful when behavior modification techniques (such as those described in this book) are not effective enough.

Progressive types of dementia, including Alzheimer's disease, affect key thought processes, including the following six areas:

1. *Memory.* A person with a failing memory may not, for example, be able to keep in mind that getting dressed and getting into a car is a sequence leading up to dinner with friends. Events begin to exist on their own, without being linked to other events. None has a larger context.

2. *Language/communication.* The ability to communicate is what allows us to connect with others in the world, to get and give information of all sorts. We rely on communication to express needs and feelings. Language is the most obvious form of communication, but there are other ways of communicating, too. We rely on gestures, body language, and facial expressions. Through dementia, the ability to communicate is gradually lost. The first problem is usually with word finding; people struggle to find the right word for the situation, such as the appropriate word in a conversation. They may forget names of people who are well known to them. Later, they may have difficulty expressing ideas; they may know what they want to say but not be able to find the words. All of this can lead to embarrassment and frustration, possibly prompting the person to withdraw. Communication difficulties and frustrations can produce emotional outbursts. Some people with the problem blame caregivers.

3. *Reasoning.* People with dementia cannot be reasonable. Most of us expect others to be reasonable, and we assume that they will be reasonable when we interact with them. Throughout daily life, we

regularly appeal to reason, and we employ logic and persuasion in many situations. And we expect others to use logic and persuasion in return. Most of all, we expect that these forms of interaction will carry the day. Dementia turns these expectations upside down. Increasingly, normal forms of interaction—like persuasion—will not work. Logic will fail and may backfire. Asking the person to think ahead through a series of steps may cause confusion, withdrawal, or impetuous behavior. As the person with dementia loses his or her reasoning power, the caregiver will need to take more control.

4. *Judgment.* Judgment is the ability we use when we ask the question, "What if?" Asking ourselves this question allows us to judge the safety, benefits, and drawbacks of a situation. The ability to imagine the possible outcomes of a situation is very important for personal safety. Unfortunately, this capacity is lost relatively early in dementia. Because of distorted thinking, judgment may be poor or faulty and utterly different from the person's previous decision-making abilities and behaviors. The person's own insight into his or her thinking problems varies greatly among individuals, and changes as the disease advances. At first, the person with dementia may be cognizant that he or she has a problem; later, he or she will not realize that there is a problem. All of this makes it hard to know whether and how much to involve the person in critical life choices.

5. *Abstract thought.* We rely on abstract thought to deal with everything in our lives that is not concrete. In fact, numerous things we take for granted are abstract. Numbers and directions are abstract, as is time. The past and the future are held in order by the power of abstraction. Possibilities are abstract, including the ability to think about the "what ifs" in our lives. Being able to know "where" and "how much" is part of abstraction, and so are relationships—the connections we share among family members and friends. Like the other powers of thought, abstraction declines with the progress of dementia. Again, this ability is lost fairly early in the disease, which means that many of the concepts we rely on to live in this world no longer have meaning for the person who has dementia.

6. *Perception.* Normal perception involves two features. First, our senses allow us to take in the world around us. Through sight and

hearing, and also through touch, smell, and taste, we take note of things outside of ourselves. Second, our brains make sense out of what we observe. People with dementia often make mistakes in sensing and interpreting things. For example, they may interpret images on television as being real and start talking back to them. Reflections, including a person's own reflection in a mirror, can be mistaken for real people who suddenly appear and disappear. Patterns in floor tile or carpets can be mistaken for holes that need to be stepped over or avoided. They may even be seen as uncrossable barriers. Such misperceptions are sometimes called pseudo-hallucinations. Since the root causes of pseudo-hallucinations may actually be situated in poor hearing or eyesight, testing and correcting hearing and visual problems can sometimes help. However, even when the person who has dementia is able to see and hear clearly, he or she may still be unable to interpret things accurately.

Frances continued on her dementia journey with her son by her side for three more years. Her activity level declined slowly over that time, and her son needed more and more help from professional care providers. Frances's physical care needs escalated, and he wasn't able to provide for all of her needs on his own.

I continue to admire the countless family care providers who step up to dedicate months and even years to caring for parents, siblings, spouses, or even nonrelatives, making sure that the person with dementia is led along a path strewn with feelings of safety, security, and love and with shared meaningful moments. Frances's son confided in me at her memorial service that although this had been the most difficult time in his adult life, it had cemented a unique bond in his relationship with his mother. He was experiencing mixed emotions: sadness at her loss, comfort that she was no longer suffering, and a strange feeling of "what do I do now?" because he also had lost his role as a full-time caregiver. Many care providers face this same roller coaster of emotions at the end of the dementia care journey, which is another reason that it's important to ask for assistance all along the way.

CHAPTER SIX

Jill

Into the Dementia Wonderland

One day at an art gallery, Jill was studying a beautiful painting of a beach, with shimmering sand, deep aqua waves, and an airy cottage with two empty beach chairs facing the dazzling blue ocean. As she stood there looking at the artist's work, she began to cry. The gallery owner came up and introduced herself, asking if she could be of assistance.

Jill replied, "My name is Jill, and my mother has advanced dementia. I am her full-time caregiver, and she seems to be getting further and further away from me as her disease progresses. The 'place' where she seems to go most often in her mind is a beach cottage she often mentioned when reminiscing about her childhood. That place seems to be very much like the place in this painting. I want to buy it and hang it in my mother's room so she and I can 'visit' this special place from her long-ago memories."

The art gallery owner was so touched by Jill's deep connection with her mother that she helped her purchase the painting on a payment plan. This simple act beautifully enriched the time Jill shared with her mother.

Lessons Learned

You will never win an argument with someone who has dementia. In fact, you may already sense that the person you are caring for will be much more cooperative if you acknowledge and give *affirmative responses* to his or her feelings and subsequent behaviors—in *his or her reality*, not in yours. This reality, from which the person who has dementia may drift in and out, is very different from your reality and from what your loved one's reality was before the dementia became an issue.

Here are two examples of affirmative responses to challenging behaviors:

1. Mr. Jones has been living in a secured memory care environment for several weeks. He keeps trying to leave through the secure door. He becomes very agitated if the care staff tells him that he cannot go out that door. He even gets aggressive with caregivers who say, "No, you can't go out this door." Care staff found the solution by redirecting him with affirming statements such as, "I am so sorry, but this door is out of order. The door in back is operating. Let me show you the way." The back door led out to the secure courtyard, and Mr. Jones could go in and out as he pleased.

2. When an adult with dementia and memory loss is asking for a loved one whom you know passed away several years ago, you are in a difficult situation. Instead of trying to bring the person into the painful reality of the loss of the loved one and causing him to experience unresolved temporary grieving, you can "reminisce" with him about the person who is no longer with him. You might ask: "When was the last time you saw her?" "How long has it been since you talked with him?" "What was your favorite time you spent together?" "Where did you first meet?"

   As you become more and more dementia-aware you may recognize that the adult with dementia who you are "reminiscing" with has passed the point of being able to effortlessly process questions and will feel less anxious if you use a simpler "feeling prompt" approach. Instead of asking "When was the last time you saw her?" try a positive feeling trigger statement such as: "You enjoyed spending time with her" or "It feels good to think about time with her." Making a statement rather than asking a question helps to "cue the person" to the feeling in the moment. It reduces the need for him to struggle with the fragmented thinking about how he might have felt or should have felt. Spend a few meaningful moments with the person affirming past memories and feelings. Most of the time he will go on to other thoughts, and neither of you will have to experience the loss and grief over and over again.

I like to relate the "reality" of the person with dementia to the notion of "reality" in the book *Alice in Wonderland*. If you are familiar with the story, you know that Alice stepped through the looking-glass mirror to another world, a fantasy "reality" she called a "wonder-land," where she enjoyed amazing adventures with the Cheshire Cat, the White Rabbit, and many other interesting characters. When she stepped back through the mirror into the reality of the parlor in her home, however, she could not bring her new friends or unusual adventures with her. They did not exist in this world.

The most challenging behaviors for caregivers sometimes are precipitated by their attempts to bring the person who has dementia into their own reality. These attempts can stir up anxiety, anger, fear, combativeness, and aggression in the person receiving care. As caregivers we can more easily connect if we confidently step through that person's "mirror" into her world and allow her to act as our "Alice"—to lead us through the dementia wonderland.

Remember: the feelings remain long after the event has been forgotten! I love the way Maya Angelou expressed this: "I've learned that people will forget what you said, people will forget what you did, but people will never forget how you made them feel."

You have probably experienced a variety of behaviors—some pleasant and some not so pleasant—from the person in your care. Although you may not be able to identify or understand the cause of the behavior at the time, you might keep in mind that there is a reason for every behavior. As the person who has dementia travels back into his past, he experiences the emotions attached to long-ago memories just as if these past events were occurring in the present. How he acts reflects how he felt *then*. In other words, long-ago emotions are influencing current actions.

If these feelings are based on memories that cause fear, anger, or insecurity, the person who has dementia will "act out" negative behaviors—for example, by resisting your requests. Your loved one or client may say or do unkind or hurtful things, or she may cry and attempt to burden you with guilt or grief. On the other hand, if the feelings are rooted in memories of joy, happiness, and security, she will tend to be kinder and more cooperative.

Additionally, the more at peace you are, the more easily you will guide your loved one or client into a place of serenity. In the next chapter, we explore further how important it is for the caregiver to be in a "happy place." The caregiver who remains calm can gently lead the person who has dementia to experience feelings of peace.

Perceptions and Approaches

Even the most challenging and bizarre dementia behaviors are born from past events. These behaviors are triggered by things that are happening now that in some way evoke a sight, smell, sound, or emotion from long ago. When you understand the root causes of these behaviors, you can put on your creative thinking cap and develop unique approaches that will help you redirect your loved one or client into more cooperative behaviors.

Even if you do not know what's causing a specific behavior, you can still use redirection to obtain a more tranquil reaction, as long as you approach each challenge from a place of peacefulness.

Family caregivers usually have no choice but to take on the challenges of caregiving. Life is suddenly interrupted. Caregivers respond in a variety of ways, but very few caregivers find that taking care of someone with dementia is undemanding, as comments like these remind us:

- "I took care of my mom for three years. It was the most difficult time in my life."
- "I took care of my wife for two years. We had to place her in a memory care facility for the last year. That was the hardest thing I've ever had to do."
- "My husband and I had so many plans for our retirement years. We were about four years away and had just started building our retirement home when he was diagnosed with Alzheimer's. We finished our home early, but we had to forget all the other plans we had. After he died, I had to sell the house—there were just too many things to remind me of those difficult years."

Remaining calm while caring for the person who has dementia can be very difficult. The stress that caregivers face is considered chronic stress because it is long term, constant, and unrelenting. This stress can be powerful enough to damage the caregiver's health and cause serious illness. Properly managing stress is vital to successful caregiving.

This chapter's message is simple: one way to manage stress is to remember that you cannot correct the dementia wonderland. All attempts to bring people with dementia into "reality" will only create more stress for both parties. Instead of setting yourself up for intense frustration, give your loved one or client *affirmative responses*. Doing so will help you remain in a place of calm confidence, which will in turn help the person who has dementia.

CHAPTER SEVEN

Natalie

Much More than Words

Natalie and George had been married fifty-seven years and had raised two sons and a daughter. When George was diagnosed with dementia and suffered a rapid cognitive decline, the family banded together to try to keep him at home. The sons and daughter were busy with their families and jobs, so most of the caregiving fell on Natalie's shoulders.

As the dementia began manifesting itself in more challenging ways, Natalie began to fail both physically and mentally. And then the level of care that George needed increased significantly, way beyond what anyone in the family could provide. George had traveled so far back into his past memories that he could not remember his children or Natalie; he began to yell at them to get out of the house. He saw his family as strangers and felt threatened by them. Finally he grew so anxious and paranoid that the family knew it was time to place him in a secured environment that could provide the kind of care he now needed.

Natalie faithfully visited George in his new home. Her visits were appreciated by both George and the staff, but George continued to revert back to a time in his past where he could not remember who she was. He would sit and hold her hand during the visits, sharing what he could of his memories as they smiled and chatted. But he would only call Natalie "the nice lady." The children also visited and were welcomed in the same way, as nice strangers.

Early one morning George made his way to the nurse's station and leaned over the counter to speak to the night nurse on duty. With tears in his eyes he told her, "Natalie came and kissed me goodbye last night." The nurse was startled, "You remember Natalie?" George smiled and shuffled back to his room. The look on his face appeared to signal that he had just shared a special secret.

Just hours earlier, Natalie had been killed in an automobile accident. At the time George spoke to the nurse, though, neither the nurse nor anyone in the memory care facility had been informed of the heartbreaking news. How did George know? Did Natalie kiss him goodnight? We will never know what clued George into sensing this tragedy.

Natalie and George's story was shared with me by one of their sons. When he finished, we wept together with tears rolling down our cheeks. It was clear how truly powerful the human heart-to-heart connection is.

Lessons Learned

When connecting to their intense past feelings and memories, people with dementia tap into a deeper level of communication. In fact, they communicate in ways that we as caregivers often cannot see or understand by normal means. People with dementia may attempt to compensate for the loss of traditional ways of communicating—such as speech—in order to understand the confusing world around them.

According to Albert Mehrabian, professor emeritus of psychology at the University of California, Los Angeles, communication with the person who has dementia is only 7 percent verbal. The other 93 percent of communication is conveyed through our tone of voice, our body language, our approach (physically moving into that person's "space" to interact), and our emotions. These signals are all "heard" and interpreted loudly and clearly by people with cognitive impairment.

As the disease strips away their language centers, people with dementia lose their ability to communicate verbally. The brain attempts to compensate for these losses by using all of the remaining senses to perceive, interpret, and acknowledge what is happening in each person's immediate surroundings. The use of other senses heightens the impact of nonverbal communication.

In summary, the person who has dementia will feel what you are feeling and reflect those emotions back.

During a training session for staff at a memory care facility, one of the residents wheeled herself into the dining room where we were conducting the training. She stopped her wheelchair right next to me. One of the staff got up and wanted to take her back into the hall, but I asked the staff member to return to her seat. I reached for the resident's hand.

The resident took my hand and looked up at me. I asked her if she wanted to join us. She smiled and said, "Yes, it feels warm next to you!" I asked her if she knew what I was feeling, and she said, "I think so. I think you are feeling happy, and I am too!"

Just before the resident came in, I had been sharing information about the importance of being in your "happy place" as a caregiver. Since the person who has dementia mirrors our emotions, if we are happy and have a pleasant demeanor, we will help the person with dementia be in their "happy place" as often as possible. This resident could feel my calm, just as she would soon begin to sense the positive emotions in all the staff who had attended the session and quickly began applying this technique.

The best way to help the person who has dementia remain calm is for you to remain calm. Do your best to leave harassed or anxious feelings outside of the relationship. Above all, take time away to find respite and keep yourself in a less stressed place. Even if you are not filled with happiness, you can still smile and make eye contact. Setting the right tone at the beginning of every interaction will result in a higher level of cooperation from the person who has dementia.

In sharp contrast to the above example, I once conducted an in-home assessment for a couple in which the wife had a dementia diagnosis. I arrived at the porch and was about to knock when I heard quite a scuffle inside. The wife was screaming at the top of her lungs, "Get out, get out, get out of my house, you b——! Leave me alone!"

I knocked loudly, and the husband answered the door looking very embarrassed. He anxiously let me in, saying, "Please excuse my wife.

She is having a very bad day and does not want the visiting nurse to take her vitals. Can you help her, Laura?"

I came around the corner to find the visiting nurse in a distressed state. She was trying hopelessly to grab the uncooperative patient's arm: "Now, you have to calm down. I need to take your blood pressure and I am late for my next appointment. You should not be calling me names. Let me get this done now. Calm down this instant!"

The wife was having no part of the nurse's pushiness and arrogance. Instead, the ninety-four-pound wife swung her tiny arms and kicked at the nurse while screaming foul words at the top of her lungs. I calmly asked the nurse if she could come back after her next appointment, explaining that I would work on calming her patient before she returned. The nurse was indignant: "She might try to hit or kick you, so watch out!" I assured her I would be okay.

As the nurse left the room, I took a deep breath, quickly surveyed the situation, and discerned that the nurse's frantic, pushy approach was a big factor in the wife's combativeness and resistance. Even in her dementia confusion, the wife sensed the nurse's frustration, which was making the wife feel apprehensive about this unfamiliar person in her house. Consider: here was a complete stranger who had come into her personal space and had been grabbing her and scolding her.

I recognized that I could help to make this agitated wife feel calmer and safe and secure only if I approached her slowly and serenely, overemphasizing a sense of tranquility as I came within reach of her and presenting a hushed, relaxed, composed, and gentle demeanor. I sat down next to the enraged woman and softly spoke as she kept up her frantic gestures and angry words: "I will go away as you ask, but I am so tired. I know that you do not want me here, but may I sit next to you and rest for just a minute? I have come a long way and need to sit in your lovely home and rest. I am soooo tired."

I spoke these words several times as slowly and as softly as I could, just loud enough so she could hear me. My words grew even softer, and she hesitated and listened. Her words also softened, and she started to relax. I took a deep breath and went quiet. Then she became quiet, and within a few minutes she fell sound asleep next to me.

When there are changes in the brain that affect memory, reasoning, and language, the primary tool of communication for the person who has dementia becomes behavior. Dementia may completely change a person's mood and personality. At first, memory loss and difficulty in thinking clearly may bother the person who has dementia. Later, disruptive behavior and other problems may start, and the person may not even be aware of what he or she is doing.

Caregiving is stressful, both emotionally and physically. Not only do many caregivers feed, bathe, and provide emotional support, but they do most of the daily household maintenance as well. According to the Family Caregiver Alliance, 22 percent of caregivers report feeling exhausted at night. Unfortunately, the more stressed you are, the more stressed the person who has dementia is likely to become. The good news is that serenity can draw out wonderfully pleasant behavior.

Perceptions and Approaches

The person with dementia is hypersensitive to what you are feeling. For example, a 2009 study by C. M. Kipps and others showed that people with dementia can no longer distinguish between verbal sarcasm and truth. Instead, they rely heavily on the feelings that come with the words. When faced with sarcasm, they will ignore any verbal misrepresentation from the speaker and will instead "read" the truth of the other person's feelings. If you sarcastically tell someone with dementia, "Oh, don't worry—I'm feeling just *fine*," he or she will probably see right through it.

My experiences have proven this over and over. The person who has dementia will understand how we feel better than they will understand what we say. If you are angry or anxious, how is the person you are caring for likely to feel? If you are frustrated and intolerant, what type of behavior will you get back from him or her? And if you are tired and burned out, how can you expect the person you are caring for to feel cooperative and helpful?

It is not only important that you care for yourself for your own sake; it is equally important to care for yourself so that you can help your loved one or client cope with this devastating disease. Since the person with dementia will mirror your feelings and moods, you have the power to set the tone. Assuming an upbeat manner will create many more positive moments for you both as you go about your day. If you can do it, you will be rewarded with an enhanced caregiving relationship.

CHAPTER EIGHT

Vada

Past, Present, and Future

One of the requirements for my gerontology degree was a delightful course called Reminiscence. Every student was paired with a skilled nursing facility resident who had been diagnosed with some form of dementia. This person was to be our "partner" for the semester.

We would meet for class at the facility and spend the first hour with our partners, getting to know them and establishing rapport and a trusting relationship. They had varying degrees of dementia, but most seemed to enjoy the attention and time that we gave them. After the first hour we would lead our residents down to a common area—the activity room—and we would all sit in a circle to participate in the group portion of class, called "reminiscence."

Each day we would have a planned theme, or topic, to spark memories and story sharing as a group. Almost everyone enjoyed the discussions of such topics as "your wedding day," "the war years," and "childhood pets."

One resident, however, did not seem to appreciate the opportunity to share. She was not showing much enthusiasm for our visits or activities. The resident's name was Vada, and her reputation preceded her.

From the beginning, the student paired with Vada had known she was in for a challenge. Vada was 101 years old and in very poor health with a terminal illness. She spoke to the staff in an abrasive way and was constantly complaining about the facility, the food, the care, and nearly every person within a ten-foot radius.

Vada was angry and anxious, and she resisted all attempts to make her last days comfortable and happy. Hard of hearing, she had loud outbursts during the group memory activity: "What are we doing here? I can't hear them. What did they say? Take me back to my room!"

This behavior went on time after time until the day our topic was "birthdays." As we went around the circle asking how people had celebrated their childhood birthdays or what their favorite birthday was, we came to Vada. To our shock, we were not greeted by the usual angry protest. In a quiet, shaky voice full of emotion, she began telling us about her eighth birthday.

She grew up poor as an only child on an isolated farm on the midwestern plains. Her father and mother worked hard from sunup to sundown, and Vada was also expected to contribute by doing loads of chores. She did not attend school. Her mother did her best to homeschool her in reading, writing, and arithmetic.

Because there were no other children nearby, Vada had few chances to play or socialize with anyone her own age. One morning about six months before Vada's eighth birthday, her mother surprised her with the news that they could throw a big birthday bash for her! Over the next six months, Vada and her mother created handwritten invitations that her father took to children throughout the county. Together they baked, made homemade decorations, and spent many days in anticipation of the big celebration.

As Vada described the preparations, her face lit up, and she related what she remembered. All of the participants in the class were mesmerized at the uncharacteristic change in her behavior, and we wanted to hear more. Suddenly, Vada began to cry, and her voice got even softer. On the day of her birthday, she jumped out of bed and ran to the window of the farmhouse. She was greeted with the sight of blinding, drifting snow. Because of the blizzard, no one could come to the party.

The pain and disappointment from years before were written on Vada's face, and the tears rolled freely. She looked around the room, "I hate being alone. My family is gone. I am sick and lonely. Please don't let me die here all alone." That was the first time as a student that I had experienced the phenomenon of a person who has dementia reliving past memories and feelings. We all rallied and did our best to comfort Vada.

At our next class, we brought her a very large stuffed bear that we had all autographed with comforting phrases: "We love you, Vada." "We are here for you." "You are not alone." She took that bear into her arms and beamed.

The following week, the staff came to our class and informed us that Vada had passed away with a contented smile, still holding her soft, furry friend in her arms.

Lessons Learned

As the short-term memory fades, a person with dementia sometimes becomes caught up in painful, unresolved memories and is trapped by the negative feelings those memories trigger. This "rut" may be the root behind unpleasant behaviors.

Many people who have dementia appreciate it when someone does something as simple as listening with a caring ear. They may express painful feelings that they are still trying to work through. When you adjust your listening skills to accommodate both the pleasant and the painful memories—listening without judgment or argument—you will become much more effective at communicating and speaking the special "dialect of dementia." This kind of listening can also create an opening for the person with dementia to resolve or tie up loose ends by working through the negative events, venting "emotional steam" that may have been suppressed for years. It sometimes even happens that the person will go back in time to escape the painful *present* reality, only to get stuck in equally painful long-ago memories.

But as we experienced with Vada, being able to share lonely and frightened feelings with other people who show true concern and empathy can help a person release those feelings and experience a more meaningful and secure life passage.

Perceptions and Approaches

When you are communicating with someone with dementia, be patient and develop a trusting relationship. Always provide a dignified and respectful atmosphere, even if the person is not always able to provide the same for you.

Each dementia journey is characterized and navigated by the person's unique personality and history, so we must provide our loved ones and clients with direction. This direction must be based upon a deeper understanding of *their distinctive courses*. Although those with dementia have much in common in terms of the disease of dementia, each individual brings a one-of-a-kind storyline, so it is up to the caregiver to listen, adjust, and change, remaining flexible and fluid in addressing the ever-evolving needs as the dementia progresses.

Sometimes the stories that the person with dementia shares will be unclear, repetitive, or even dull. However, the more time you take to show genuine interest—intently focusing on what the person can share with you about his or her past—the better able you will be to build a deep connection. This connection will, in turn, help you develop care solutions that effectively meet the social and emotional needs of your client or loved one.

Vada is a prime example. Because our class was able to hear her story and heal her wounded heart, we were able to give her the compassion she needed before her passing.

Human beings, including human beings with dementia, need to be able to express their feelings to someone who cares; this is especially true of strong (and perhaps unpleasant) feelings from one's past. The strong feelings that are directly connected to past memories do not magically evaporate as we age. On the contrary, they often come back late in life to haunt us, just as we observed when Vada relived the agonizing sentiments associated with her eighth birthday. By listening for and catching an emotion that may have been bottled up inside someone for years, we allow the person to express those feelings and ease their minds and hearts.

CHAPTER NINE

Joe

Communicating the Gift of Value

Recently I was asked to consult at a local skilled nursing facility to assist with a new resident who was being very uncooperative. He would not allow the staff to guide him to the dining area for meals or to his room for sleep, and he was exhibiting a puzzling, repetitive behavior. I will call this dear fellow Joe.

When I arrived, the staff led me to a long hallway where I saw Joe shuffling along and feeling the hallway walls, reaching as high as he could and as low as he could, muttering to himself as he studied the spot of wall in front of him. Up and down the long hall, back and forth he went. When the staff would come alongside and ask him to come for lunch, he would give them an emphatic "No!" and go back to his task with complete focus.

He made no attempt to converse with the staff, and there were no family or friends we could talk with to find out what might be causing his unusual actions, so I asked to see his chart. The chart gave me an idea of where he was in his past reality.

Utilizing a tool called *reflective action*, I stood very near to him and began to "mirror his actions" as we moved together on the wall. I moved at his pace and did exactly what he did. Then after a few moments, I stopped and touched the back of his hand, moving directly in front of him and taking both of his hands in mine. I looked into his eyes and asked him, "Joe, do you see this? Someone has done a very poor job on the finish of this wall. We need to get our best repairman here to refinish it. Who would be the best man for this job?" He looked intently into my eyes and answered, "Frank!"

I quickly asked him, "Where is Frank?" He still had his hands in mine as we both turned our heads this way and that, visually searching for Frank. When it was clear that Frank was not immediately at hand, I looked at my watch and said, "Oh, it's lunchtime. Frank has taken his usual lunch break. Let's go get our lunch, and we can get Frank to fix this wall first thing this afternoon."

Joe took my outstretched arm and shuffled down to the dining area. I sat with him while he ate lunch and told me about his work.

The staff asked, "Laura, how did you get him to do that?"

I replied, "I simply visited Joe in his past memories of his occupation, as a creative and artistic wall finisher! He was a specialist as an Italian wall finisher, a craft he learned from his father and brought over to our country when his family immigrated here. He is beautifying and fixing your walls for you!" And as soon as he was done eating lunch, off he went, back to "work," visiting a place that gave him feelings of pride and self-worth.

A few weeks later, I called to follow up and was pleased to hear that this technique worked well for ongoing cooperation whenever the staff felt it was needed. The staff had even gone a creative step further! One evening as it was getting late and a staff member was attempting to get Joe to his room for bed, she encountered some resistance. She told Joe that if they requested help from Frank at this late hour, they would probably have to pay him overtime. Joe's eyes widened, "Oh, no! No overtime!" He immediately followed her to his room for the night.

And Joe gave another *affirmative response* when the staff implemented a successful plan every day at lunchtime. A staff member simply brought him his lunch in an old-fashioned metal lunchbox. He would carry it to the dining room and oblige the staff by calmly consuming his meal with little or no resistance. The old lunchbox triggered images of his past noontime routine, giving him the sense of security and familiarity he was searching for.

Lessons Learned

If you were confused about your surroundings, could not remember who the people near you were, felt disoriented and overwhelmed and could only access memories and feelings from your distant past, where would you go to feel the most secure and content? Of course: back in time, to memories that brought you happiness, delight, and feelings of self-worth and purpose.

In contrast, if you had frightening or unhappy feelings driven by painful memories, you would naturally want to avoid those unpleasant stops on your journey. However, as we saw with Vada in the last chapter, the person who has dementia may become "stuck" in those negative unresolved memories and feelings. Understanding the person's behavior helps reveal whether he or she is experiencing pleasant or unpleasant memories. If someone is experiencing negative feelings, we want to affirm the person and yet bring comfort and peace to the situation. Conversely, when the person is in a good place, we want to help reinforce the positive memories and feelings.

Remember: you will never win an argument with a person who has dementia. But whenever you affirm the emotions that the person is experiencing, you will instead enjoy a magical connection! Affirming emotions will provide many wonderful opportunities for you both to feel appreciated. Joe's story illustrates how we all respond in an affirmative way when we are directed toward positive feelings. Making people with dementia feel valued helps create an emotional safe place for them to land amidst their confusion.

The brain and the memory-storage processes are extraordinarily complex. They are made up of several distinct parts, and every part has its own function. While the storage part of the brain has separate functions in and of itself, all of the parts of the brain must work together to complete even the simplest task. As dementia affects each area of the brain, certain functions or abilities can be lost, and the brain will then attempt to compensate for the loss, desperately trying to make sense of the ongoing confusion. When one or more dots in the connect-the-dots schematic are missing, the person is in need of help or a coping mechanism to complete even a common or familiar task.

Further, changes in behavior and changes in the person's inability to communicate may be related to damage caused by the disease. He or she may experience many bewildering feelings but not have the ability to express them verbally.

Perceptions and Approaches

Our usual ways of communicating become less effective as the dementia progresses. Communicating effectively with a person who has dementia requires skill, confidence, and adaptability. Approach each situation with patience. Repeat phrases that produce an *affirmative response*. Slow down, watch, and listen—and repeat, repeat, repeat. Use creativity to express both your feelings and your message. Practice these new skills to convey your message effectively and to feel confident when you handle each difficult situation.

Look back on how we connected with Joe. Through *reflective action*, we mirrored his physical actions and showed him that we were on his side and working to enter his world rather than bring him into ours. After that, the door was open to communicate with him verbally.

When you want to communicate with your loved one or client, be sure to get the person's attention and make eye contact. Make certain the person feels that he or she is your only focus. Look him or her directly in the eye and be totally present. Speak slowly and clearly, giving only one message at a time. Limit outside distractions such as a TV or radio.

Use actions as well as words—the old "show and tell" skills that you learned as a child in school. For example, if you are going out for a walk with your loved one or client, hand the person a sweater and point at the door at the same time, saying that it is time for his or her walk.

Even when their communication abilities are failing, you can still show people that you understand their unique attempts to get across what they wish to share. Watch facial and bodily responses. The person's reaction to what you say can give you an idea of how much she understands. Respond to his or her moods and emotions, especially when the words do not make sense or are inappropriate.

And finally, never lose sight of the importance of nonverbal cues. We all communicate by emotion, expression, and touch. Holding a hand, or smiling when talking, can convey much more than any words.

We all want to be heard, validated, and valued. The following story beautifully illustrates how important it is to bring value to the person who has dementia.

Lessons from Hazel
By Deana Chitambar, RN, CHPN

The many facets of my job as a hospice registered nurse include teaching a class on Alzheimer's disease at dementia care facilities. My students are professional caregivers who are responsible for assisting residents with activities of daily living (ADLs), such as dressing, toileting, and bathing.

One day in class, we were having an interesting discussion on the definition and diagnosis of Alzheimer's disease. Discreetly entering the back of the room, the facility's director brought in a resident named Hazel, who did not want to stay seated in her wheelchair. Because Hazel was at risk for falling, it was apparent that the wheelchair was a safety precaution, so one of the student caregivers was asked to care for her during our class time. The caregiver stationed herself next to the resident, and the class discussion resumed.

It wasn't long before Hazel was out of her wheelchair and trying to escape from us, however. The student caregiver would get Hazel seated in her wheelchair only to find her a few seconds later scrambling back to her feet. While we clearly needed to divert her attention from trying to leave her wheelchair, she was obviously on some sort of mission. I decided to put into practice a technique that I had recently learned from Laura Wayman's caregiver training.

I started by introducing myself to Hazel, and then I calmly and politely asked her where she was going. She explained that she had to leave because she wanted to start her new business.

With those words, she had given me the opportunity to enter into her dementia world and demonstrate to the class the affirmative response method of communication. I shared with Hazel that we were holding a meeting regarding new businesses and would like to have her sit down and join us. Immediately—and with great enthusiasm—she sat back down into her wheelchair, and we were off to a great start!

With the rest of the class sitting with us, I asked Hazel about her upcoming entrepreneurial venture. She told us that she wanted to open a baby store to supply products to her clients. I involved the class in Hazel's dementia wonderland by guiding the students to discuss what might be stocked in a store like the one Hazel had in mind and how she might price the items. While giving these affirmative responses to Hazel, I continued teaching. I used this opportunity to demonstrate how important it is to get to know the residents they care for, and how much they need to relate to the residents' worlds. It was exciting to see how well the principles I had learned from Laura really worked.

My encounter with Hazel reminded me of a very important lesson. The main focus of providing care for the elderly, especially those who have dementia, is not about my agenda (like teaching a class), wanting someone like Hazel to sit back down in her wheelchair, or even my feelings. The focus is on the needs of the elderly person in front of me. The interaction with Hazel reinforced the idea that if I am going to be able to respond to the immediate needs of a person who has dementia, I must be willing to enter into his or her world attentively, respectfully, and without argument. Most importantly, I must treat each person with genuine loving care.

CHAPTER TEN

Lucy and Betty

Thinking Outside the Box

It came as a shock to the family when Grandma Lucy was diagnosed with Alzheimer's. The 87-year-old was always so bright and loved to be involved in her children's lives, spending hours with them and the grandchildren whenever possible. She never tired of sharing remarkable stories from her rich, long history. She was an attractive lady, taking immense pride in her appearance, even wearing matching shoes with every outfit.

But Lucy began to struggle emotionally. She also suffered the common losses of dementia—short-term memory malfunction and a breakdown in information processing. Her diabetes brought on major health complications. Finally, the family had to make the tough decision to place her in a memory care facility.

A mere two weeks after Lucy had settled in and was apparently making a smooth transition into her new home, the diabetes caused circulatory failure in her legs and set off a dramatic chain of events. Everything culminated in the unfortunate medical necessity to amputate both of her legs below the knee. After a long hospital stay and a brief time in rehabilitation, she was back "home" in the memory care facility—now in a wheelchair. But this time she did not make the transition smoothly.

Lucy returned with a disturbing behavior that was puzzling to her family, the staff, and the other residents. She would spend her days rolling around in her wheelchair from one resident to another, shaking her finger and yelling that they had stolen her shoes. Lucy would call out for the staff to "get her shoes back from that thief," angrily accusing everyone in her path. The staff would quietly assure her that no one had stolen her shoes and would attempt to bring her into reality by gently reminding her of the necessary but heartbreaking surgery and loss of her legs. This approach only escalated her paranoia, emotional distress, and anger. There seemed to be no way to calm or comfort her.

The staff and family consulted me for advice. After talking with Lucy's family about her past and the most recent events, I asked the daughter to tell me about Lucy's favorite pair of shoes.

Her daughter said: "Mom had so many pairs of shoes that it's hard to know which ones were her favorites. She did have a beautiful pair of red satin pumps; they were very stylish in her day, and she would often wear them to church or on special occasions. She even asked for them right after she moved here, before her surgery, but we did not want her wearing them because they have a very tall heel, and she could have easily taken a bad fall."

I asked the daughter if she would bring that pair of shoes to her mother. She looked bewildered and said they were packed away, but she would. When she brought in the shoes the next day, we all stood back as she handed them to Lucy. What happened next brought tears to our eyes. Lucy's face lit up, and she got a big, bright smile reminiscent of a child's on Christmas morning. She stroked the shoes, turning them this way and that to view every inch. Then she put them in her lap and rolled off in her wheelchair to proudly flaunt them to the other residents. She did not seem to mind that she could not wear them, only exhibiting utter satisfaction as she carried them everywhere in her lap. That night, the staff placed them on her nightstand in plain view, and Lucy relaxed and went to sleep.

The next day and from then on, she continued to contentedly carry, display, and admire her beautiful red shoes.

Betty loved living independently. She was a private person, enjoying time for herself in her home of forty-seven years. She had raised her only child, a daughter, in that house and would pass the time tending to her lovely garden, full of prize-winning roses. She would also spend countless hours sitting in her front porch swing, keeping track of the comings and goings in her neighborhood. Alert and curious, she would hear all, see all, and delight in telling all to her daughter whenever she would visit, passing along the gossip of the day about her neighbors.

That is, until she developed dementia. As Betty's abilities decreased, she needed more and more help with day-to-day tasks in her home. Betty's daughter lived only a few minutes away and recognized that she needed to balance the losses her mother was experiencing with her remaining abilities. The goal was to allow Betty to function independently and to enjoy living in her home as long as possible. She would watch her mother closely and step in and assist with care only when she truly needed help.

One of the difficult challenges the daughter had to face was letting Betty know it was no longer wise for her to drive. Betty's eyesight had deteriorated significantly, and her reaction times had slowed. She was not a safe driver. Her daughter now provided all of the transportation, organizing errands and shopping trips around her own work schedule so that Betty could keep her doctors' appointments, excursions to the beauty salon, luncheons with her friends, and grocery or shopping trips every week. This routine also gave the daughter an excuse to visit regularly, check on Betty's nutrition and medication needs, and help out with small chores and daily tasks.

But as the dementia progressed, Betty became more and more resistant to getting up and out of the house on time, especially for her appointments. On those days, the daughter would arrive in the morning a couple of hours before the appointment and find Betty still in bed.

"Time to get up, Mom!" the daughter would cheerfully exclaim, "Today you have an appointment with Dr. Smith at ten a.m. I'm here early to help you get ready. I'll go start the shower while you get up." Betty would sit up drowsily, look around and say, "Where do we have to go today?" The daughter would say it again, "Today you have an appointment with Dr. Smith at ten o'clock. Rise and shine!" Betty would lie back down and say, "I didn't sleep at all last night. Could we go another day?"

Already the daughter could feel the recurring frustration brewing.

She had reminded her mother about this necessary appointment at dinnertime the day before. But the predictable and tedious routine was happening anyway. It was getting more and more difficult for the daughter to disguise her emotions, and her negative feelings showed through in her facial expressions and demeanor.

Betty was picking up on the frustrations but could not remember asking the questions and repeating herself, so she had no way to understand why her daughter was upset. It was all very confusing. With great concern and hesitation she asked her daughter again, "Where are we going?" With all her might the daughter attempted to stay calm: "You have a doctor's appointment in an hour. We have to hurry to get there in time."

I listened to the daughter explain the frustrating circumstances. She felt like a terrible daughter and caregiver for getting so annoyed with her sweet mother. She said that she knew her mother could not remember, but it was still so difficult to keep reminding her every five minutes without going absolutely batty. And it felt like the harder she pushed Betty to cooperate and hurry, the slower and more resistant Betty became.

After getting to know Betty and her past likes and dislikes, I worked with her daughter to come up with a new approach. Happily, it worked like a charm. By reframing her approach only slightly, the daughter received the gift of an affirmative response. An added bonus was that the whole experience became meaningful and fun instead of tiresome and repetitive.

This is how it went: "Good morning, Mom, time to get up. I'm here to take you to your doctor appointment at ten o'clock. How did you sleep?"

Betty replied as she usually did, "I didn't sleep at all. Could we reschedule for another day?"

"No, Mom, but we can get you back here mid-morning to rest after the appointment. I'll go get the water started for your shower, but first I want to tell you a secret about your neighbor, Mrs. Jones." The daughter launched into a juicy story she made up about one of her mother's neighbors and then said, "Come get into the shower, and I'll tell you the rest."

Betty's eyes lit up, and her face was bright with interest. She stepped into the bathroom and listened intently to the "gossip" that her daughter conveyed. She was even cheerfully cooperative as she dressed, and her new, accommodating manner continued all the way through breakfast, the drive to the doctor's, the wait at the doctor's office, and the trip home.

As her daughter related the "gossip," Betty provided appropriate commentary: "Oh my goodness," "I'm shocked," and "I can't imagine!" The daughter reported that it was the best time she'd had with her mother in a long while! And from then on, this approach worked like magic!

Lessons Learned

The techniques employed with Lucy and Betty are called *creative interventions*. A creative intervention involves simply finding a clever way to meet the specific needs of a person who has dementia. Lucy wanted to hold her bright red shoes, and Betty loved gossip.

In developing your own creative interventions, you will find they work best if you have the opportunity to research and collect information from the individual's past. Each person with dementia has a unique and long history of joys, sorrows, pleasure, and pain. Tapping into the significance of historical events that make the individual feel loved, secure, valued, or safe will usually bring those feelings to the present time and allow you to share in the origins of the feelings attached to a memory. The better you come to understand the person for whom you are caring, the better able you will be to provide his or her care.

Alzheimer's disease and other forms of dementia progress over time, affecting how the person functions on a day-to-day basis. As you learn about the changes the disease causes, you will develop realistic expectations of the person's abilities.

In the early stages, ask your loved one or client how you can help him or her stay independent and maintain a sense of control. It is best to encourage independence as much as possible, since doing so will reduce the burden on you and on the person for whom you are caring. As the dementia begins to hinder the person's memory and abilities, he or she will find it beneficial to contribute to self-care, even if it is in a small way.

To a point, independence boils down to the old saw: use it or lose it! Of course, later in the disease the person may well not be able to participate in his or her own self-care.

Perceptions and Approaches

A common tip from experienced caregivers is to *learn to be patient.* Granted, this is not always easy, but it will pay off in rich rewards. Do not rush people who have dementia. Give them plenty of time. Although it is often faster and easier to do things for other people rather than wait as they perform tasks for themselves, allowing them to complete basic tasks gives them a sense of value. Help them to feel proud of even the simplest accomplishments.

Above all, be sure to continue your favorite activities together. Listen to music. Take a walk. Talk about your favorite shoes. "Gossip" about the usual suspects. Focus on the person's talents and abilities. Look for common interests and use them to establish communication connections.

No matter how the disease affects the individual, it is important to treat him or her with dignity and respect. Although certain abilities will be lost, the person's emotions and feelings will remain, as will the need for companionship and belonging. To add to the person's quality of life and help him or her maintain a unique identity, provide activities and interactions that bring a sense of joy and celebration.

Never lose sight of the person who was there before the dementia.

CHAPTER ELEVEN

Edna

You're Just Imagining Things

One afternoon a middle-aged woman named Sue called the home care company that I was managing. Sue was her Aunt Edna's closest kin, but she lived several hours away from her aunt. When I picked up the crisis line, Sue explained the situation in a panicked voice. "Aunt Edna lives alone in a large house and has been doing okay until recently. Now I'm worried because this morning she called me and said I had to come to her house right now and get the clowns out of her living room."

You can imagine how Aunt Edna's plea sounded to her niece. Apparently, these "clowns" had kept Edna up all night, telling her they had come for the clothes she had taken from them. They would not leave her alone, and Edna was very afraid. The niece wanted to know if our company could provide a caregiver to stay with Edna and make sure there were no "clowns" who were causing this torment.

She explained, "Edna is threatening to call 911 to get the police to take out the clowns. There are no neighbors nearby that I can call on, so can I hire someone from your company to sit with her until I get there?"

I told the alarmed niece that I could do an emergency assessment within the hour and find out more about the situation. Then I would call her back and let her know if we could get a caregiver to help out until the family could make other arrangements.

When I arrived at Edna's house, she greeted me warmly at the door and immediately let me inside. I explained to Edna that I had experience in dealing with clowns, as well as other foolish visitors, and that in the past I had been successful in getting similar folks to leave the premises. Edna looked at me with incredible relief. "Last week I called the police," she sighed, "and they simply told me there were no clowns. They left me alone with them."

She was thankful that I believed her and that I wanted to do something to solve the problem. I use open-ended questions to help people with dementia guide me through their wonderland, which helps me understand their perception and reality. It is important to begin each question with "who?" "what?" "where?" "when?" or "how?"

"Where are these annoying clowns?" I asked her. Edna pointed to a large sofa. Sighing with frustration at my lack of awareness, she said, "All three of them are right there, as you can plainly see." I watched her face and realized that she could indeed see clowns sitting right there in front of us. To her, they were very real.

So I walked over to the sofa where the "clowns" were camped out and said in a firm and confident tone: "What are you here for? I need to ask you to leave now!"

Edna piped in with a condescending tone in my direction, "They want their clothes back. I already told everyone that."

Continuing to face the clowns, I asked Edna, "Where are these clothes?"

Edna led me down the hall to her bedroom and her overstuffed clothes closet. I asked her to hand me the items of clothing that she believed were the ones the clowns were asking for. Without hesitation, she handed me several brightly colored items out of her closet. I asked her if this was all of them. Edna nodded, and I carried the clothes out to my car.

As I exited the house, I looked over my shoulder and said to the nonexistent clowns, "This is all of it. I will take you and the clothes back to where you belong, and you must never come here again and bother this nice lady." (The clowns were indeed "nonexistent" in my reality, but Edna's behavior showed they existed and were very "real" in her dementia wonderland.)

I put everything in my trunk and went back inside the house to let Edna know I would take care of this matter and that she had nothing to worry about. I also told her that I had a coworker who was coming right over to keep her company until her niece arrived. Edna seemed grateful and calm; resolving her problem had made her feel safe and secure.

The caregiver from our company arrived a few minutes later, and for several months she came to stay with Edna on a regular schedule, at the family's request. Edna never again claimed to see or be bothered by clowns. Our office quietly returned the brightly colored clothing back to Edna's closet without incident.

Lessons Learned

Unfortunately, as individuals struggle to cope with dementia, paranoia like Edna's is not uncommon. People with dementia may have misperceptions or hallucinations about family members, old friends, and strangers. In most cases, this is just a phase that eventually subsides, but there is no way to predict how long these symptoms will last. The severity of the symptoms can depend on the type of dementia.

The resulting behaviors are especially related to a loss of control. As people with dementia come to rely on others for assistance, they may feel as if the caregivers are taking over their lives or even robbing them. And as the dementia progresses, they often lose the ability to recognize that they themselves might be to blame for missing items. For example, they might store some valuables away to protect the items from theft and then forget where they hid them. It would then seem to them that the misplaced items must have been stolen, and they will often accuse the people closest to them of stealing the items.

If a person with dementia still lives in his or her own home, the most likely target of the accusations will be the family or professional in-home caregiver—or possibly a housekeeper or landscaper. In a care facility, such as an assisted living or memory care community, the main target generally will be the care staff, other residents, or even visitors. You may hear statements such as these:

- "A man came here and he took my jewelry."
- "That woman stole my scarves, but she says she didn't take them."

Instead of reacting to these behaviors, coping with and managing them is the key to making the person feel safe and supported. Imagine what it would be like if you suspected you were being followed home by a strange car one evening, thought you had been receiving odd or threatening phone calls, or believed you saw someone hiding outside your bedroom window. Now imagine that you shared your fears with your family and friends, and that even though you were genuinely scared, they calmly dismissed your anxiety as foolishness. How would this make you feel?

Perceptions and Approaches

As noted in earlier chapters, it is best not to argue with a confused person. Disagreeing may only escalate and fan the fires of anger, anxiety, paranoia, and fear. If you cannot win the battle, change the war. No matter how outlandish the claim or accusation, listen and proceed as though you believe everything the person with dementia is saying. Plan to take action that will give the person a sense of relief. The most frustrating response she can get from you is an argument to try to convince her that the situation is not real. Although in this instance it was helpful for me to ask Edna questions, because she still could process this information and give me answers, keep in mind that as the dementia progresses, it becomes more and more difficult for the person to respond. A dementia-aware caregiver uses fewer questions and gives fewer options and instead takes positive action and makes simple statements. The more you "think" for people with dementia, the kinder and more supportive you are in their eyes. Short and sweet, less is best, fewer words and more action. Agree, agree, and agree some more! This change in your care approach as you become more and more dementia-aware will bring you much relief, as well as helping the one you are caring for experience more moments of calmness and peace.

This is a big change in how we have always communicated with adults, so it takes practice! I even have to remind myself to ask less and do more, as this is a core component of dementia-aware communication. For example, when you first greet someone you often ask "How are you?" You expect a common response such as "Fine, how are you?" I have observed how this ordinary and simple question can make the person with dementia uncomfortable, stopping them in their tracks as they struggle to process an answer. When I began to notice this was causing some difficulties, I changed this customary greeting to a positive statement such as: "You look great today!" or "It is so nice to meet you!" The change in their response was remarkable, so much more relaxed and less confused. I now make it a habit to communicate more and more often in this manner, starting from the first moment I spend with the person who has dementia symptoms.

Many of the things that people with dementia do are attempts to empower themselves by hanging on to the remaining elements of control and choice they still possess. As we go through life, we suffer diminishing control over many things. These losses put dents in our emotional armor, especially if they are caused by dementia. Examples include loss of

- memory
- knowing where you are and who other people are
- physical health
- relationships
- independence, such as the ability to drive or to take care of personal finances
- the ability to care for the basic needs of daily living, such as bathing, eating, grooming, toileting, walking, or even standing up

It is vital to allow people to retain a sense of control as far as you and they are able:

- If Mom feels secure when she has a credit card and checkbook (even though the accounts are closed), then let her have them, even though you are now in charge of the finances.

- If Dad keeps claiming that someone is poisoning his food, perhaps what he means is that the food tastes very different. He may fear that the food is somehow a cause of his confusion and loss.

Given all of the other losses that persons with dementia may be experiencing, the last thing they want to feel is that they have lost their grip on reality. When people with dementia insist that the people around them affirm their perception of the world, they are actually asking for help in framing their own worlds. By providing validation, you will help to make everything else seem less confusing to them, even if the relief is only temporary. Your affirmation provides a brief respite, allowing the person with dementia to rest his or her mind in the midst of what must feel like constant chaos.

Remember that each situation and scenario is very real and true to your loved one or client in his wonderland. It must be very frightening to experience events that seem so real and then not receive validation from others. As you listen to and focus on every complaint, accusation, or angry outburst, try to allow yourself to be open to what is being said. Being open will let you develop steps to solve the person's challenges, just as you would tackle real problems. Be a detective and discover the who, what, when, where, and how of each situation. Handling your loved one or client's issues is yet another way to bridge the gap between the two of you and enter into the dementia wonderland. And if helping "get the clowns out of the house" will bring the person with dementia to a place of calm, then get creative and do what it takes.

The restlessness and anxiety that accompanies the person with dementia on a daily basis can be overwhelming. As noted in earlier chapters, there is always an underlying reason for the person's behavior— generally a feeling or memory from the past that is causing confusion, fear, anger, paranoia, or aggressiveness in the present. Sometimes the person may be searching for someone or something, not even knowing who or what it is she is looking for. Worst of all, the person with dementia does not know how to resolve or calm the constant sense of tension and frustration. Having the caregiver believe what the person is saying may be the only key to peace and serenity.

As you approach each situation with an open mind, also consider the possibility that a person's behavior may not be totally rooted in dementia. For example, the paranoia caused by dementia may be exacerbated by sensory impairment.

I once heard a story of an elderly man who continually told his family that the president of the United States came to visit him. The family would upset this gentleman by arguing with him that this was not possible. Then one day the son walked into his father's room when the presidential debates were on TV. The father had impaired vision and was hard of hearing, and the TV was blaring in the background. The gentleman was not hallucinating or telling stories; he had poor eyesight and difficulty distinguishing between what was real and what he was hearing on the television. He truly believed the president was in the room with him.

Throughout the dementia journey, all you can do is your best as you face the challenging role of caring for your loved one or client. You may be able to count up the many things that you feel you have done wrong, but the fact is that we are all human and make mistakes. Take time to find a little magic in each day and celebrate the small wins along the journey.

When your loved one or client is affected by dementia-related paranoia, he or she may make some very hurtful accusations. Even though you are making tremendous sacrifices to take care of her, she may angrily look you straight in the eye and say things like, "You stole my purse! I know it was you!" These kinds of comments hurt, and they may be devastating, even triggering your own past wounds and conflicts. If you are a professional caregiver, there may be the added fear of losing your job when the person with dementia makes accusations of theft. In these instances, be sure to communicate with your manager or supervisor. Additionally, you may need to have a meeting with the person's family to discuss the situation. Whether you are a professional caregiver or a lay caregiver, let these situations be powerful reminders of your own need for self-care.

As frequently as possible, look for easy ways to lighten your load. Lock the bathroom door and soak in a bubble bath. Get together with your friends and play cards. Take a walk or read a book. Watch the latest ballgame or a comforting movie. Choose your favorite relaxing activity. You need to have a place where you can remove stress and emotionally vent.

In addition to practicing these quick fixes, schedule time for long-term stress management and maintenance. Longer-term stress busters can include attending regular caregiver support groups (the local chapter of the Alzheimer's Association can provide lists of support groups in your area), seeing a counselor who is experienced in care-provider stress issues, or learning meditation or progressive relaxation exercises. There are also wonderful training programs that are specific to stress management and that are suited to both family care-givers and healthcare professionals.

One such program that is currently receiving rave reviews is called HeartMath. HeartMath training programs, coaching, publications, licensing programs, and innovative technology may help people live more rewarding and healthy lives—personally and professionally. I have not tried these training programs myself and mention them only as an example of the kinds of programs that are being developed.

Early in my own dementia-care journey, I worked alongside a local medical hypnotherapist who professionally recorded relaxation and mood-enhancing CDs. These CDs contained soothing music that helped me reduce my own stress and provided a calming environment for the people with dementia whom I was working with, as well. Many CDs with calming music and words are available through bookstores, libraries, and online.

Some in-home care providers and dementia-care facilities use a program called Snoezelen Therapy, which is designed to assist in calming people with dementia who are agitated. Snoezelen Therapy utilizes a "relaxation room" that consists of fiber-optic lighting fixtures, aromatherapy, soft and changing environmental mood lighting, comfortable seating, and relaxing sounds and music. By engaging as many senses as possible, this atmosphere may create a sense of safety and security. Again, I have not tried this program with my clients.

Whether you are a family or professional caregiver, during these tough days and moments I encourage you to do whatever it takes to manage your stress level. This includes the time-honored practice of asking for assistance. Attending a support group will help you find out what other caregivers have done to cope with the bizarre stories, unfounded accusations, and paranoia that the person with dementia may exhibit. To further educate yourself, attend an educational conference, seminar, or workshop. It is imperative that you protect and safeguard yourself from the potential negative impacts of this disease.

CHAPTER TWELVE

Margie

If You Keep Doing What You Are Doing . . .

The daughter of a German woman and a U.S. soldier, Margie grew up in postwar Germany. We can only imagine what her childhood was like. We do know that she and her family spent a year in a tuberculosis ward. Her father, a military cook, was often away, and Margie ended up caring for her mother, who suffered from depression, as well as for her sister, who was targeted by bullies at school because she was deaf (a result of meningitis). Although Margie was mentally and physically abused by her mother and was often battered in scuffles while defending her sister, she maintained a positive outlook on life. Eventually, her family moved to America.

Years later, in 1968, Margie met Pete, a sailor based at an air station in Maine. The following year they were married. Margie and Pete enjoyed an amazing marriage and had one child, Jennifer. Eventually they moved to California and ended up in the foothills above Sacramento.

In 2007, Pete began noticing worrisome signs in his wife. Though she was still relatively young to be diagnosed with dementia, she had increasingly noticeable short-term memory loss and struggled to recall things that had never been a problem in the past. Both of Margie's parents had died of Alzheimer's disease, so Pete and Margie were familiar with the symptoms. Pete was proactive and consulted with their family physician. Margie was diagnosed with early-onset Alzheimer's dementia.

This was the beginning of a long and difficult downward spiral. In the months following the diagnosis, Margie got confused and turned the wrong direction at the end of their driveway, backing into a tree. She would also get lost driving to familiar places within a short distance of home.

To make matters worse, she began to have frequent bouts of anxiety and paranoia, with the result that she wandered away from home. Several times, Pete was forced to ask the local police for help in bringing her back safely. On Margie's fifty-eighth birthday, she went to church with her husband and wept uncontrollably throughout the entire sermon. Afterward, to Pete's dismay, she refused to get in the car. Extremely agitated, she started walking, and Pete followed her closely in the car. Then she waved down a passing car and got in, driving off with perfect strangers. Fortunately, they drove her right back to church. Pete followed, but she again refused to get into his car.

From there she took off on foot and disappeared. It was the police who found her standing in front of a nearby Catholic church. Margie remained adamant about not leaving with Pete, so he called their daughter, and Margie agreed to go home with Jennifer for the time being. Pete was so shaken by the unfortunate situation that he had to be admitted to the hospital for extremely high blood pressure. He was experiencing the stress-related physical strain of caregiving for a memory-challenged adult. Pete came to the painful realization that he would have to get Margie additional care from another source.

Margie was placed in a memory care environment, but she did not adjust well. After a brief hospital stay, she was placed in a skilled nursing facility. But this particular institution was not proficient in managing the type of dementia behaviors that Margie exhibited, including anger, combativeness, and anxiety. The situation went from bad to worse.

When the staff called Pete to discuss his wife's severe behavioral problems, Pete contacted me for help. He explained that she had pushed, hit, and kicked a male caregiver who had tried to assist her with a shower. And this was not the only incident. When she was acting out in her fear and anger, she would even threaten other residents.

In what would become a cycle, after an episode of combative behavior the staff would send Margie to a hospital for a mental health assessment, and the hospital would send her back—over and over.

Unfortunately, this type of situation is common in facilities that do not properly train staff with the communication tools to gently and lovingly redirect the person with dementia. I agreed to spend a few hours with Margie at the facility. My plan was to then approach the facility staff with some training solutions so they could more successfully manage Margie's agitation and aggression.

When I arrived, Margie was in the activity room with a group that was playing a game. She sat at the table with the other residents but was not engaged at all. After a few minutes, she stood up. Most of her waking time was spent walking around and around the hallways. In fact, she slept very little and rarely sat still.

Her daughter, Jennifer, introduced me to Margie as a friend of hers. Pete was also there and gave Margie a kiss on the cheek. She smiled at both of them and said hello to me. We chatted as we walked together and sat for a few minutes in the lobby. It was apparent that Margie felt uncomfortable sitting for any length of time. Pete explained that she had back pain, and I wondered if this was one of the reasons she was constantly on the move. After forty-five minutes of visiting and walking, I recognized it was time for a staff member to change Margie. She was incontinent and needed to be cleaned up. As we passed the nurse's station, I discreetly requested the change. The male nurse asked me to take her to her room so he could send someone to take care of her personal needs.

Her room was long and narrow, with three beds and curtains to section off each bed area for privacy; hers was at the very back. As we entered, Margie's calm and pleasant demeanor instantly changed to suspicion—to that of a frightened victim. She became nervous and looked at me with sudden distrust. As I turned to go back out into the hallway, two male caregivers marched in to change Margie.

They moved with determination toward her and pulled the privacy curtain. In less than two minutes, Margie came bursting into the hall with her pants unzipped and her face bright red with rage. She was screaming and cursing, vowing that she would never go back there.

She made her way to the nurse's counter, picked up a pile of books and a book stand, and pitched them at the nurse behind the counter. Pete and I came up beside her and, as calmly as we could, talked to her and stroked her arms. This was a method that always worked for Pete when he needed to calm her from an agitated state. Jennifer was then able to walk her down the hall and further quiet her.

I asked the nurse in charge if they had female staff available to change Margie, since it was obvious that she was very frightened by the male care providers. I was told that they were unable to fulfill that kind of request due to difficulty scheduling enough female nurses to cover every shift. Moreover, they needed to send caregivers strong enough to "hold her down to change her." Pete, Jennifer, and I were astonished. We reminded the nurse that Margie had not exhibited aggression in the hospital or with female care providers.

However, we were ultimately met with a refusal to modify the approach. The saddest part of this story is that after the next time Margie was taken to the hospital, the nursing facility refused to take her back, stating that they could not manage her care and that her behavior was too difficult for them to handle.

It has been said that insanity is doing the same thing over and over and expecting a different result. In this instance, the facility staff's inflexibility made it impossible for them to care for Margie adequately.

Lessons Learned

Research is showing that some relatively basic interventions that do not involve pharmaceuticals can be used to ease behaviors. A simplified approach to managing agitation can be summed up as "modify the environment, modify the behavior, and medicate as a last resort." While most of this research was conducted in residential facilities and nursing homes, family caregivers can follow the same principles.

In our professional caregiving training sessions, we always tell the care providers, "If you keep doing what you are doing, you will keep getting what you are getting." And if what you are getting is not an *affirmative response,* try a different approach.

All types of behavior are forms of communication. When a person with dementia acts out, he or she is trying to tell you something. Agitation is often the result of the inability to deal with stress, pain, or fatigue. The key is to identify whether the behavior is related to a specific event or whether it stems from a sudden or unusual environmental stimulation that causes an emotional outburst and then escalates into a combative flare-up:

• An *event-related cause* could be an unpleasant situation involving necessary care, such as when a caregiver attempts to clean the person up after an incontinence-related accident. The care receiver may strongly feel that his or her privacy is being invaded by a stranger. The event may even bring up memories from an abusive past event.

• *Environmental stimulation* that causes agitation could involve, for example, moving the person with dementia from home into a hospital-like skilled nursing facility. It may be that the person feels bereaved because he or she associates the hospital setting with a memory of the loss of a loved one.

Either of these kinds of memory stimulations—which are usually innocent—can trigger unpleasant, seemingly bizarre, or even dangerous actions on the part of the person with dementia.

Take note of patterns and subtle clues that tension is mounting. The more proactive you are in redirecting the behavior before anxiety escalates, the more successful the redirection will be. Avoid telling people with dementia "no" or "you can't" or trying to physically prevent them from going somewhere or doing something. This could be perceived as aggression, and they will feel they must forcefully protect themselves. The tendency toward aggressive behavior often increases at the end of the day as stress and fatigue build.

Perceptions and Approaches

What are some ways to deal with agitation?

I have enjoyed great success using music with which the person with dementia is familiar. Playing calming music or the person's favorite type of music can lead to a decrease in agitation. Use this tool before and during meals, since it can increase food and fluid consumption. When relaxing and calming music is used during bathing, it can make the person with dementia less resistant to personal care. Use the music familiar to those growing up in the '30s, '40s, and '50s. Try everything from soothing classical music to hymns and spirituals or big band tunes.

Light exercise each day can also help to maintain function of limbs and decrease problem behaviors. Going for a walk—preferably one to two hours before dinner—several times each week may help reduce pent-up agitation in a healthy, productive way, as well as stimulate the appetite. And besides, exercise is good for *you*, the caregiver, too.

Activities that include social interaction are also helpful. Sometimes large groups and many strangers are not well received, but a companion or volunteer who consistently spends one-on-one time with your loved one or client is usually welcome.

Additionally, never lose sight of the person who was there before the dementia. Activities that reflect your loved one's previous life or career are very effective. And everyone can derive pleasure from the simplest activities. You can reminisce, converse, or sing together.

Above all, a serene approach *from the caregiver* is the magical key to successfully managing agitation. The person with dementia is ultrasensitive to your moods and feelings and will mirror back whatever is felt from the person providing care. So check your anxiety, agitation, and stress at the door before you spend time with a person with dementia.

CHAPTER THIRTEEN

Harry

It's Bath Night!

Born and raised in Denver, I grew up in the beautiful state of Colorado. My father's father, Harry William, who was born in England, immigrated to the United States at the young age of 13. He came through Ellis Island, worked hard, married, and raised two children, one of whom was my father, Jack. When Harry retired, he built a small log cabin in the picturesque village of Red Feather Lakes in the Colorado Rockies.

I was the youngest of five siblings, and our family also had many foster children. Every summer, we would all spend several weeks at Grandpa Harry's cabin. The mountain slopes provided ample space to run, climb rocks, fish, catch frogs, and dig for worms. We would also ride the wooden horses that Grandpa had built out of logs, have fun in the playhouse he had built with his own hands, and make popcorn in the cabin's fireplace.

The cabin had no running water or electricity and the fireplace was effectively the central heating unit. When we needed water, Grandpa Harry would haul it from the well. Needless to say, we children managed to get rather dirty while playing in our mountain paradise. Now that I think about it, we probably did not smell particularly good, either.

However, Grandpa Harry had a once-a-week routine for cleaning up that he had brought with him from his younger days. When we visited him, we were treated to the same time-honored tradition of the Saturday night bath. Grandpa would heat up the bath water on the wood-burning stove in the kitchen, then pour the hot water into the big aluminum tub. We all took turns, oldest first, in the progressively dirtier and colder water.

Since I was the youngest, I always got the coldest and dirtiest water! At the time I didn't mind, but as an adult, I still remember the cool water and not being able to see the bottom of the tub through all the grime from my older siblings. There was not a shower or a bathtub with running water in sight, and I am positive that if we had asked Grandpa about taking a shower, he would have looked at us as if we were speaking a foreign language.

Taking showers, especially seven days a week, is a tradition that belongs to later generations. In my grandfather's day, water was a precious commodity and bathing was a major production: clean water had to be hauled in and heated and dirty water had to be hauled out. Baths happened once a week. Daily cleaning-up consisted of a sponge bath. This "bird bath," as my mother called it, involved a bar of soap, cold water, and a clean rag or sponge.

Lessons Learned

Many people who have dementia resist personal-care tasks like bathing. When caregivers ask me to help them overcome this reluctance, they often tell me the same story: they ask the care recipient whether he or she wants to take a shower, and the response is a firm "No." "I just took one," he might say, or "It's not time yet." Or the person might stare blankly, as if she doesn't understand the question. Once I was providing care for a family friend whose father reacted to bathing by crying in the shower. He repeated over and over that it was too hot or too cold and pleaded with me to stop or to hurry up and finish. It was an unpleasant experience for both of us. Sometimes the topic of showering obviously makes the person who has dementia feel afraid, a response that makes me wonder why the person is having such an extreme reaction to a common daily task.

To solve this mystery, we must remember that people who have dementia travel back into their pasts, retrieving old memories and feelings. They tend to seek those memories that make them feel secure, safe, and happy. The language of dementia and each person's unique dialect come from long-ago traditions and events. They also rely on all five senses: sight, hearing, smell, taste, and touch.

Bearing this in mind, we can explore whether the word *shower* means the same thing to the person who has dementia as the word *bath*. What memories might be brought to mind by a shower? Water hitting him in the face, for example? Or might a bath bring to mind easing her toes into the water to test its temperature? Was the room where he bathed as a child a cold, tiny space with glaring white tiles and bright lights, or was it a lantern-lit kitchen in a farmhouse warmed by a cozy fire? Were the sounds of bathing harsh and echoing, or were they the familiar voices of family members? Was their family very private, or were others allowed to wash and touch sensitive parts of their nude bodies?

Now imagine what it would be like to experience a shower in an unfamiliar place with strange people around you.

Perceptions and Approaches

It's no wonder that caregivers frequently face resistance to the common task of bathing. A sensitive approach may make all the difference. When your loved one or client resists letting you help him or her with a shower, avoid saying the word *shower* or *asking questions*. Instead, try simple and positive action statements:

- "It's time to clean up now."
- "Let's go take our bath before the water gets too cold and dirty."
- "I am so hot, a cool bath would make me feel better. I'm going that way, so come and give me a hand getting the bath ready."
- "A warm bath sounds so good. It would warm you down to your bones."
- "Your daughter called and said she is on her way to take you to —— [the doctor's office, lunch, etc.]." Use whatever topic might motivate this person to get ready.

- "It's Saturday. Time for bath night!" Draw on the person's past routine, if you know what it was. Use terms that are understandable within the person's dialect of dementia.
- "I picked up your favorite lavender-scented soap. You smell so good when you use it. Let's go use some right now."

If the approach is not working now, come back and try again at a time when he or she is more likely to be cooperative. If Mrs. Smith is not a morning person, approach her in the afternoon when she is in a better mood.

Bathing an elderly person who has dementia in a traditional bathtub is difficult and dangerous, so you may want to give the person a shower, even though you call the undertaking a "bath." You need to make the routine as familiar as possible, however. If there is a shower bench, have the person sit down; this is generally safer anyway. Use a handheld adjustable showerhead. It can be startling for anyone to be suddenly hit in the face by running water, so start by washing the feet and work your way up. Move slowly and with confident purpose. Talk in a quiet and reassuring tone. If you are nervous or rushed, the person will pick up on it and feel the same way.

Here are some more tips to make each bathing experience more peaceful and cooperative:

- Make sure the setting is quiet and private, with adequate but not overly glaring lights. A stark or bright light can feel cold and institutional. Honor the need for modesty; hold up a towel or undress and redress the person as you go. It is always appreciated if you provide assistance while keeping the person's dignity in mind.
- Be prepared. Have everything that is needed at hand: soap, towels, brush, etc. If you get the person ready and in a cooperative mood for bathing, you do not want to miss the window of opportunity because you have to go fetch a towel. Furthermore, it is not safe to leave the person alone, especially if he or she is wet and soapy.
- Give instructions *one* at a time. Do not rush the task. Keep in mind that the person's ability to process information has

been slowed and interrupted by the dementia, so keep everything simple.

- Demonstrate the task at hand. A demonstration sometimes prompts the individual to begin the task himself or herself. For example, the person may begin to comb his or her own hair by watching you comb yours. Remember to always allow the person to do whatever he or she can. Do not focus on what is no longer within the person's abilities; encourage the person to do what he or she is capable of. Even a small sense of accomplishment feels good.

- Consider your own attitude and appearance. What is important? If it turns out that your loved one or client can tolerate a shower only once or twice a week—with a sponge bath every day in between—consider this a small compromise in the whole scheme of caregiving. If the person is not incontinent, the shower and sponge bath rotation usually provides adequate personal care. Most likely it will also become a familiar and comforting routine. As you take care of your own hygiene regularly, it sets a good example for the behavior you desire from your loved one or client. Even though people who have dementia may not be as aware of their own hygiene, they will still evaluate yours. It is not uncommon for ladies from prior generations to be critical of other women who venture out in public without full makeup and a fine hairdo. Older men who used to pride themselves on their fitness have no verbal filter and may tell people point-blank when they need to lose weight.

- Play soft music, preferably the style that is the person's favorite. When the person is in his or her "happy place" and enjoying music, he or she is more likely to be cooperative. Additionally, praise and compliments always help, just as noted by the old saying, "You can catch more flies with honey than you can with vinegar!"

- Finally, some caregivers have found that promising care recipients a bowl of ice cream can work wonders as an incentive.

As dementia causes the more recent memories to disappear, many memories from the past begin to feel more and more like now. When you are bathing the person who has dementia (or performing any other difficult care task or activity of daily living), frame your approach in a way that is familiar to the person. Doing so will help you enhance communication with the past feelings and memories where the person now resides. By using common memorabilia or topics from the past in your conversations, you can build the necessary trust. In a world of handheld electronic devices, instant communication, and fast food, we do not think in terms of the technologies that were used in the early twentieth century. Many of these gadgets have become impractical, but what is obsolete to us in a practical sense could be a gold mine for fostering great conversations with the person who has dementia, forming bonds as we enter into that person's world of fond memories.

Items of nostalgia can be used to redirect your loved one or client to a sense of familiarity and security, especially if they have a special meaning to the person you are caring for. For example, a person who worked for a long time as a secretary would relate to a manual typewriter. Someone who enjoyed church music might like to talk about the old pump-style church organ, or a homemaker, about the wringer-style washer or party-line telephone. Discussing these items can help you develop a social history that is customized to the person's past individual experience. Here is a list of such items to consider talking about when working with your loved one or client. You may be able to show the person some of these items or give them to him to handle (or keep!).

- party lines on the telephone, along with a crank or rotary-dial telephone or a telephone operator who heard all the community's gossip
- pump-style organs to accompany the church choir
- wringer washing machines and washboards
- coal heaters or stoves, with the familiar coal bin and coal chute to the basement
- toilets that flushed with a chain

- pedal-driven sewing machines
- manual typewriters
- cars that started with a crank in the front
- glass milk bottles delivered to the door by a horse-drawn cart or truck
- the Good Humor ice cream man
- doctors who made house calls
- glass Coca-Cola bottles in a wooden carrier
- bottle caps lined with cork
- the malt shop on the corner
- a juke box
- penny candy
- S&H green stamps—filling the books and buying items at the stamp store
- sock hops, poodle skirts, and the jitterbug
- the Charleston and flappers
- the Iron Curtain and fallout shelters
- live radio shows, such as *Walter Winchell*, *Jack Benny*, *The Bickersons*, or *The Shadow*—with one sponsor and its famous slogan "You can trust your car to the man who wears the star"
- favorite vintage TV game shows:
    - *Beat the Clock*
    - *Concentration*
    - *I've Got a Secret*
    - *Truth or Consequences*
    - *What's My Line?*
    - *You Bet Your Life* (a.k.a. *The Groucho Show*)

Take the time to talk about these and other long-ago memories. The person you are caring for was probably greatly influenced by at least one if not many of the subjects on this list. The more you discover about your loved one or client's past, the more easily you will be able to reach her through her unique dementia dialect.

You will probably encounter days when things go smoothly and other days when they do not. The person with dementia has mood swings like everyone else. Just stay on course, and be willing to be flexible in your approaches. If bath time does not get done this morning, try the afternoon or tomorrow.

For more tips on successfully conquering the common struggle of bathing a person who has dementia, you may want to read *Bathing without a Battle: Person-Directed Care of Individuals with Dementia*, by Ann Louise Barrick and coauthors. Like its popular predecessor, the second edition of *Bathing without a Battle* presents an individualized problem-solving approach to bathing and providing the personal care for individuals with dementia. This edition includes historical material on bathing and substantially updates the section on special concerns, which includes pain, skin care, identifying the appropriate level of assistance, transfers, and the environment.

CHAPTER FOURTEEN

Susan

Dealing with Disruption

❧ ❧ ❧

With Alicia Murray

Susan had finally accepted the promotion she had worked so hard for over her entire career. She had been offered the job numerous times in the past, but she had turned it down because her children were still little and the position demanded longer hours.

But now she was up for it! And she was finally the manager of her own department at the age of 42. She felt this was a new chapter in her life, and she was enjoying the rewards of her expertise and dedication.

Then, one day, her cell phone rang. Her heart dropped as she heard the voice of her sister, who rarely called unless there was an emergency. Perhaps her sister was calling to congratulate her on the promotion: "Hey, Sis, what's going on?"

"Susan, you need to get down to the hospital right away. I think Mom may have had a stroke!" Their mother, confused and agitated, had been found wandering down the middle of the street. Her speech had been slurred, and she had been walking with an unsteady gait. Not knowing what to do when she got the call from a neighbor, Susan's sister had dropped everything and rushed her mother to the hospital.

The next four hours in the hospital were agonizing, as Susan and her sister tried to get information from the doctors. It felt like they were in the ultimate boxing championship and were losing badly. Then they finally got the answers.

Susan's mother had had a series of small strokes, and her sudden change in behavior was caused by vascular dementia. The doctor suggested she stay overnight for monitoring and also recommended placing her in a rehabilitation center or taking her home and getting professional caregivers to assist her. The doctor told both daughters that the mother they had known and loved was still in there but was now presented in a different package. She would probably not remember a lot of things, and she would also need twenty-four-hour care because her strokes had affected her memory and judgment and left a portion of her left side paralyzed.

Susan and her sister went to a nearby diner to talk over what needed to be done for their mother. Since their father had died a few years earlier, their mother had lived on her own, not wanting to go into one of those "old folks' homes."

To complicate matters, Susan's sister, who was quite a few years younger, had just gotten married and was planning on moving out of state the following month. Her husband had been offered a new position with his company, and she had been transferred within hers. They had already sold their home and were living in temporary housing until all the paperwork for his job came through. She offered to help pay for a caregiver for their mother but thought it would be more economical if their mother moved in with Susan rather than going to a care facility. Susan agreed that she could save money by hiring a professional caregiver during the day but taking care of their mother herself at night. The sale of their mother's home would help raise money for the caregivers.

That night, Susan called to get pricing for many different in-home care companies. Making the calculations, she figured that if the caregiver was there for six hours a day, she and her older kids could manage the rest. So she made arrangements for an in-home caregiver to work at her house five days a week for one month.

That month was far more difficult than anyone could have imagined. Susan constantly got phone calls at work from her mother. Her mother said that she did not need a caregiver and insisted that she could move back to her own house. The phone calls, with the same conversation, kept coming every couple of hours. Her mother would tell the caregiver that she was going to lie down for a nap, and then she would sneak off to call Susan, over and over again.

Susan knew she could not keep this up. Her boss had already talked to her about the excessive personal phone calls and the amount of time she had taken for doctors' appointments, suggesting she take some time off to figure out another solution. Susan had many projects due on a deadline, and she worried that a temporary leave of absence would jeopardize her career. But she could not stop the phone calls and she could not rearrange the doctors' appointments for after work.

What was she going to do? Not only were her newfound opportunities slipping away, she was also physically exhausted. Plus, the family was in an uproar over the disruptions that the changes had caused. And if she lost her job, the financial implications would spell disaster.

Lessons Learned

Susan is one of many caregivers trying to juggle the daily responsibilities of work and caregiving. Attorney Todd C. Ratner, who specializes in elder law and estate planning, notes that sixteen million Americans find themselves sandwiched between two generations, struggling to raise kids while caring for an aging parent and holding down a full-time job. This multidirectional tug-of-war can be the leading cause of stress in family caregiving. Overwhelmed and unable to meet the constant demands, many caregivers tell us, "There's just not enough time in the day!" And it is so difficult to ask for help.

Well, I cannot make the days longer, but I can help make the days easier. When I started working with Susan, she was very upset and frustrated with her mother's challenging behaviors—not only the phone calls that would not stop, but also the late night wandering and the same questions repeated endlessly. Susan, her family, and her job were all suffering.

I asked Susan to buy a tape recorder and record short messages that the professional caregiver could play for her mother throughout the day. The caregiver would introduce the recordings by telling Susan's mother that Susan had left a message on the answering machine: "Hi, Mom! I wanted to let you know that I'm in meetings all day, but I'm thinking of you and will call back later."

This little trick stopped the excessive daily phone calls. Every few days, Susan would re-record the messages and add different stories that her mother could reminisce about. It relieved some of her mother's stress and allowed Susan to focus on her job. Susan also started having the daytime caregiver take her mother to her doctors' appointments. Susan would follow up with the doctor by telephone to discuss her mother's health. Now she could get a full day's work done.

She also enrolled her mother in an adult daycare program through the local hospital, giving her three days a week out of the house. Susan realized that she needed to access as many of the senior community resources as possible. Asking for assistance from friends, family, neighbors, professionals, and the community did not make her a failure after all!

Susan joined a caregiver support group that met in the evening one day a month. By sharing her struggles with others who had similar challenges, she learned that she was not alone. Every three months, Susan's entire family, including her children, were invited to a meeting devoted to family matters. These meetings were designed to develop a team spirit, empowering everyone as they discussed the difficulties that filtered down to even the youngest child. They also promoted proactive approaches to caregiving. The family gained a clearer understanding of dementia and learned tips for sharing more meaningful moments with Susan's mother.

Above all, Susan realized that she had to take care of herself, or she would eventually burn out. She focused on eating right, exercising, and squeezing in extra time for activities she enjoyed, like taking a hot bath and reading her favorite novels. Getting restful sleep became a high priority. She made sure to thank all of her supportive coworkers. A few of them had their own heavy family responsibilities, and they agreed to ease the burdens by helping out with each other's projects.

After six months, Susan's mother developed some serious health problems and had to be placed in a skilled nursing facility that could provide her the medical care she needed. The family knew they had pursued every resource to help keep her at home as long as possible.

Perceptions and Approaches

Many of the caregivers who attend my presentations share their own stories and experiences. A common theme among them is the tension that caregiving puts on their entire families, not just on the person who is the primary caregiver. Caring for a person with dementia can put strain on even the most well-balanced family.

There are disruptions in schedules, meals, family events, and personal space. The family's finances can also be adversely affected—even drained—not only because the family is paying for private professional care, but often also because family caregivers must change jobs or take on additional jobs to work around their new roles. Because the person with dementia requires so much care, young children and teenagers often don't get the time and attention they need. And this disruption may happen just as the children need more of their parents' time, for one reason or another. The emotional toll on everyone can be extreme. Before taking on the daunting challenge of caring for a relative with dementia in the home, family members must anticipate what this will mean in terms of the day-to-day dynamic and factor that into the decision.

To cope with the challenge, you must access all of your options for support, including local community resources. Never be afraid to ask for help. Asking for help is a necessary part of your caregiving role. If you are able to maintain an open-minded approach to problem-solving, you will feel more effective and you will be less stressed.

Grace

Moving beyond Guilt

With Alicia Murray

Grace was a very active woman. She loved to go to church, take pottery classes at the local community center, and spend time with her husband, Ned. He was her confidante, her soul mate. When Ned was diagnosed with Alzheimer's, there was no option in her mind other than to become his devoted full-time caregiver.

Ned's diagnosis was heart-wrenching. Grace talked about the emotions that crashed around her: the grief of knowing there was no cure, the loneliness of missing her partner and friend, and the anxiety of knowing he would not be with her much longer. Taking care of her husband now took her entire day. She no longer attended her pottery class or went to church. She felt that she had to be there with Ned every minute.

Grace was exhausted. Further, she had completely isolated herself from the outside world. Family members offered to help her, but she always turned them down. Like so many other caregivers, she felt guilty asking someone else for assistance to do something that she truly believed she ought to be able to do herself.

With Alzheimer's disease, memory loss and challenging behaviors become more noticeable as the disease progresses. Grace was working harder and harder to redirect Ned's activities. Getting him to do simple things—things that in the beginning stages of the disease he had been able to do with just a little help from her—now required a lot more effort. Grace also began to have her own health issues.

The family had to intervene, and they called me for help. As Grace and I talked about her situation, she realized that she was on a destructive path and that she needed to make changes to preserve her own health. She made a list of all the family members who had offered to help, and she called them to set up a schedule when they would come and sit with her husband. Grace began attending church on a regular basis again, and she signed up to take her favorite pottery class.

She also joined an Alzheimer's support group, where she could talk with family caregivers who were in the same situation she was in. Grace found the support group to be very helpful. Because there were family caregivers whose loved ones were in different stages of dementia, she learned from some of them and taught others what she had learned from her own experience.

The caregiving journey is full of lessons. For Grace, giving the gift of experience to other caregivers was the ticket to relieving her feelings of guilt and working through the new and sometimes difficult emotions she struggled with. Best of all, once she was relieved of guilt, she was able to share many more meaningful moments with her husband.

Lessons Learned

Grace's story brings us to an extremely common caregiving emotion: guilt. Guilt is remorse for having done something wrong. But would it have been wrong for Grace to ask for help in addressing her own needs? Did Grace have to feel guilty about taking one hour a day for herself? Should she feel guilty about needing a break from her caregiving duties? The answer is obvious: *no.*

Grace was a wonderful wife who had taken on the caregiving role and had not thought twice about her own needs. But guilt keeps family members from doing things for themselves, and not doing anything for themselves leads to physical, mental, and emotional stress and, possibly, breakdowns. Many family caregivers feel guilty as a result of being faced with one of the hardest jobs they will ever do. They feel guilty if they have fun. They feel guilty if they leave their loved one home alone or with someone else. They feel guilty that they cannot do it all. Guilt sneaks in on these family caregivers regardless of how effective they are or how much time they spend doing this job. This guilt becomes a thunderhead on a sunny day, clouding one's judgment and cultivating sadness and even depression.

Perceptions and Approaches

Unjustified guilt is destructive in many ways. Perhaps its worst aspect is that it makes you as a caregiver believe you are a failure, when in reality caregivers are the heroes and leaders in the face of dementia. To help you cope with the guilt and any other strong emotions you are experiencing you must first understand this concept. Then you need to find out what's causing your feelings of guilt, talk about your feelings, and take time for yourself.

Caregivers heap undue pressure on themselves and feel guilty about things they do not need to feel guilty about. Moving past guilt can be hard, but you owe it to yourself to find freedom from it. As Dorothy Womack has written, "Release the guilt you carry and listen with your heart—you will truly find [that] your loved ones not only dwell in peace, but wish the same for you as well."

CHAPTER SIXTEEN

Virginia

Laughter Is Therapeutic

🌿 🌿 🌿

With Alicia Murray

Virginia was a full-time caregiver for her mother, who had dementia. One morning, Virginia was cooking breakfast when her mother came into the kitchen complaining that her pants were too tight. Virginia turned around from the stove to see what her mother was talking about and nearly burst into laughter. Her mother was standing there with her legs through the sleeves of her blouse, trying to pull them up past her knees.

Holding it all in, Virginia gave her mother an *affirmative response* without making her feel silly or stupid for trying to put on a blouse the same way she would put on a pair of pants. She guided her mother back to her room, taking full responsibility for the shrinking pants by explaining she must have washed them in hot water and shrunk them accidentally. She helped her mother get dressed and then assisted her to the table. While her mother was eating breakfast, Virginia sneaked into the bathroom and laughed so hard she had tears rolling down her face.

🌿

Lessons Learned

Sometimes it can feel like there's not a lot in your life to laugh about. But laughter is a wonderful stress buster and has great effects on your body. In fact, it increases blood flow, decreases stress hormones, boosts metabolism, and helps put our problems into perspective. Most importantly, it can help us keep our sanity in overwhelming situations.

Perceptions and Approaches

Think about what you can do to bring laughter into your life. I enjoy spending time with my family and friends. The young children in my family are full of laughter, and hearing their pure joy never fails to bring a smile to my face.

Even watching a funny show or movie with your loved one or client can be therapeutic. One woman told us a story about the time she spent caring for her mother. Her mother's favorite show while growing up was *I Love Lucy*, so the daughter bought the entire collection. They would spend a couple of hours a day laughing together, and she explained that those moments would forever stay within her heart.

Translation: Start laughing now! I hear many caregivers say, "I'm sure I'll be able to laugh about this someday." The sooner you quit waiting for "someday," the more you will enjoy your caregiving role today.

Sometimes people with dementia say and do things that are funny, like Virginia's mother's shrinking "pants." *Give yourself permission to laugh today.* Find humor in a difficult situation, if you can. Your caregiving role may be hard, but each day is precious, so take time to enjoy the moments that you share. As comedian Bob Newhart reportedly said, "Laughter gives us distance. It allows us to step back from an event, deal with it, and then move on."

CHAPTER SEVENTEEN

Beatrice and Henry

The Power of Gratitude

Beatrice and Henry had been married for many years. After the children were grown and the house was empty, Beatrice realized she did not really have a lot in common with her husband.

She thought he could be a bit overbearing, and she did not like how he laughed at things that were not at all funny. She was extremely bothered by the way he read his newspaper in the morning at breakfast, while slurping his coffee and clanking his spoon in his cereal bowl. Just being around him made her sick. She talked with her friends about Henry and all his annoying habits and how life was not what she had imagined. She spoke of divorce, but one of her friends, who had been through a couple of nasty divorces, told her that Henry was a good man and that she should see a counselor before seeing an attorney.

Determined either to seek help or to see an attorney, she went to the counselor recommended by her friend, but not without skepticism, and with anger in her heart. She asked herself, "How can this counselor help me?" As she slouched on the couch and told the counselor why she was there and the frustrating things that her lovely Henry was doing, the counselor began to smile. "Beatrice, I have an assignment for you," she said. "I want you to go home, and every day I want you to tell Henry about something that he does that you are grateful for. It has to be something new every day. It has to be honest.

And it has to be done for the next two weeks. Then come back and see me again."

Needless to say, Beatrice was thoroughly upset. She had gone to the counselor to get either a solution to the situation or permission for a divorce—not to get a homework assignment. The next morning at breakfast as Henry slurped his coffee and rattled his newspaper, Beatrice rolled her eyes. "How am I going to find something about him that I am grateful for?" She stood at the counter in the kitchen staring at Henry eating his breakfast when she noticed his nails were very nicely groomed. She said to him, "Henry, I am very grateful that you always take such good care of your nails." Small but honest: she only had to think of thirteen more and she would be home free.

The next morning the gratefulness was not overflowing as she stood at the counter in the kitchen racking her brain for something she could say to Henry. Then, like a light switch being flipped on, she noticed his tie. What a nice tie that was—he always matched his ties to his suits. "Henry, you always have the best-looking ties. They always match your suits so nicely." Henry put down his newspaper, smiled, looked down at his tie and said, "This is the one you gave me for my birthday."

The next morning was a little easier. Actually, she had spent the remainder of the previous day thinking about what she would say, and before Henry could pick up his newspaper, she blurted out, "You always take such great care of your shoes. They are always so shiny and clean." Henry smiled and replied, "You look lovely today. Is that a new outfit?" Beatrice smiled and affirmed that it was.

The following days were amazing; the breakfast table had become a place where they had conversations instead of eating in silence. The compliments had become bigger and more personal. The time they spent together had become richer, and Beatrice was remembering who she had fallen in love with years ago.

When she went back to the counselor for her two-week appointment, the counselor was delighted with the progress Beatrice and Henry were making. The counselor explained that sometimes people take the little things in life for granted, only seeing the glass half-empty. But when you change your perspective and search for the things to be grateful for, you begin to appreciate those little things that have been overlooked.

Three months later Beatrice and Henry were celebrating their second honeymoon.

Lessons Learned

It is hard to remember how important it is to be thankful for everything we have in our lives, especially when we are faced with the daunting task of caring for a loved one or client who has dementia. Research shows that caring for someone with dementia is three times harder than caring for someone with a physical ailment.

It may be difficult to find something to be grateful for, but it can be even small things like, I'm grateful I have clean sheets or a roof over my head or shoes on my feet. In my training workshops and presentations, people often come up to me after class and say that they did not believe they had anything to be grateful for—but that they are surprised at the power of appreciation when they list even the little things.

Perceptions and Approaches

When working with people with dementia, look for the good in the situation. It can be the simple fact that when you visit them in their world, they are more cooperative. That is something to be thankful for, and especially if you are a caregiver who has been thrust into this position involuntarily, cooperation is a huge blessing.

By changing our perspective and focusing on the positive instead of the negative, we are able to see things more clearly and are often able to appreciate the importance of the time shared with others. We also understand just how important it is to ignore the unimportant cobwebs in the corner of the house.

If you develop the daily habit of writing at least five things you are thankful for in a gratitude journal, no matter how small they may be, you will find that it gets easier and easier to exist in a place of gratefulness. The end result will be positively dramatic!

If you keep a journal, you can also track changes in your loved one or client, identify any potential causes of resistance or combative behavior, and adjust your strategies accordingly. Further, if you meet with other caregivers, your journals can be excellent resources and help guide all of you as you share lessons learned.

You may feel you need the support that comes from sharing your thoughts and feelings with others. Some days you may need an empathetic ear, someone who will listen and will not judge. Other days you may need a safe place to vent. Friends and family are a great place to start.

As other caregivers in our stories have discovered, a support group can give you a place to talk with other caregivers who understand the disease and know exactly what you are going through. Meeting in a group will give you an opportunity to share your own experiences, get practical suggestions that can help you, and experience the joy of helping others as well. A support group can also help you manage stress and feel less isolated.

As you proceed through your caregiving experience, recognize that you may be going through a variety of emotions, including frustration, fear, and sadness. These emotions are normal and common among caregivers, and they may come and go. Sometimes caregivers even get depressed. The person with dementia and other family members may be experiencing the same types of emotions, too. If your feelings or those of your loved one are overwhelming and persistent, do not hesitate to talk to your doctor and ask for help.

Remember, you are not taking this journey alone. And keep in mind that there can be joy and fulfillment along the way.

CHAPTER EIGHTEEN

Sean

The Puzzling Pieces of Grief

With Denise Pedersen

The following story is an account of how a dear, lifelong friend of mine came to devote her life to being a certified grief recovery specialist.

Sean was my firstborn child and only son. He was born when I was just 21, a child myself. As I held him and looked into his beautiful blue eyes, he brought great joy into my life, and through his birth, I saw the miracle of God for the very first time. Three and a half years later I gave birth to Sean's little sister, Danalyn. From the moment Sean laid eyes on her, he beamed with pride. The relationship they shared was the most rewarding gift of my life, and as the years went on, they continued to grow closer and closer.

Since I was a single mom for many years, the three of us developed an extraordinary and unique bond. We spent many hours talking, laughing, playing, and growing up together. My children are my life and my heart.

On Sunday, September 19, 2004, Sean was on his way home after a late night of being out with friends. He never arrived.

On Monday morning, when I realized that Sean was not in his room sleeping, which would have been the norm, Danalyn and I knew that something was not right and we started making phone calls. Sean absolutely loved to be at home, and it was unusual for him to stay at a friend's house. Besides that, he would have contacted us.

When night came on Monday, we called the police, and the search began. For eight days, we looked almost twenty-four hours a day to find him. We organized search parties and had a search dog; we even had a helicopter. We made thousands of calls. It was like living in the Twilight Zone.

On the ninth day at 1:30 in the afternoon, we got the call that no parent or loved one is prepared to receive. Sean had been found dead on a heavily traveled interstate freeway near Sacramento, California. He had fallen asleep while driving and veered off the road, crashing into some trees and a sound wall. Sean had been ejected from his car and was hidden behind such dense brush that neither he nor his car could be seen from the road.

From that day on our lives were forever changed, and Danalyn and I began to understand the definition of the word "grief."

I was in shock. I was unable to think clearly or make decisions, let alone follow through with any decision I had made. I was numb and could not figure out how I was going to continue to live without dying of a broken heart. I turned to a few local churches and counselors, and while everyone wanted to console me, no one knew how to give me the help I desperately needed. Because I was unable to find any kind of support system that met my needs, I began listening, reading, and learning as much as I could about grief and how other people have survived this nightmare. Along the way, I learned many things that I now attempt to share with others when they ask for help.

I also decided to take my broken heart and reach out to other families that had lost a child. I have been doing this ever since. Focusing on others helps me to know that I am not the only one who is hurting. For those who have suffered a loss, grieving is a journey through which we will have to travel for the rest of our lives.

But there is hope. With grief professionals and friends to pray, support, and encourage each other, we can find comfort this side of heaven.

Lessons Learned

Through this tragedy, my friend, Denise Pedersen, has found a way to allow something meaningful to come from a heartbreaking situation.

I have witnessed firsthand Denise's truly unbelievable courage and compassion.

On many occasions, I have been asked to support grieving caregivers during the final stages of the dementia journey. Through Denise's story, I realized I could learn how to help caregivers deal with the conflicting emotions that come with loss. By sharing her journey, Denise taught me that people's grieving experiences may have many similar emotions but that every grieving experience will be unique, with different facets and pieces.

Each facet and piece needs validation and compassion. Although grief can be a confusing puzzle, the grievers themselves are not broken. They do not need to be fixed. They need to be heard and to have the freedom to feel and understand their emotions in a safe environment. Grief is an individual, scary, and unknown path that cannot and should not be pushed, blocked, or changed. The needs and pace of the griever should be honored.

As Denise says:

> When we suffer great loss, the first step is to allow ourselves to feel the pain. We excel at intellectualizing everything, telling ourselves things like "He or she is in a better place" or "We must keep busy" or "Time heals all wounds." Sometimes those proverbs can be comforting. At other times, they sound great on paper, but knowing or thinking them does not make the loss less painful; it only makes us hide the pain from ourselves and from others. And bottling up pain leads to physical, emotional, and relational problems.
>
> Often when we are experiencing deep pain, we isolate ourselves from family and friends, which compounds the sadness. Instead, it is much healthier to acknowledge that the tragic situation feels horrible and that we do not know how we are going to continue.
>
> The next key step is to find someone to talk to, namely someone who will not judge, analyze, criticize, or try to fix us. Look for a person who will calmly listen and validate your feelings of pain, anger, and so on. If we do not find a safe

listener, we will risk turning into a pressure cooker with no one to loosen the lid and release some steam.

When we find good listeners, we become better listeners ourselves. During our own journeys, it is therapeutic to help others who are traveling down this lonely path we call grief. In helping others, we find that we are not alone. We meet people who are further down the road toward healing, giving us hope that it is possible to continue living. We will also meet people who are newer on this journey, reminding us of how we felt in the first few minutes, days, weeks, and months after our loss.

Keeping our loved ones' memories alive is also beneficial for the healing process. Think of what they loved to do and create memorials in their names. For example, if they loved to garden, plant some flowers in memory of them. Play their favorite music. Celebrate their birthdays, anniversaries, and other days that were special to them.

Bear in mind that we cannot compare our grief with the grief of others and that we must not minimize our loss. If we downplay our emotions, we will not be able to fully feel or acknowledge our pain and loss, and that will leave us unable to help others who are in a similar situation. Anticipated loss is just as painful as sudden loss. No one can say whether losing a newborn child is harder than losing an aging parent, or whether losing a spouse is harder than losing a sibling. Even though the deaths and the relationships we had with the people are all different, we need to know that grief is grief, pain is pain, and loss is loss.

If you are a caregiver assisting someone with dementia, you are losing your loved one a piece at a time. You will have to continually grieve each loss as it is presented: your loved one's loss of physical abilities, loss of memory (including when he or she forgets who you are), and loss of ability to carry out everyday functions. At the same time, you will be grieving the loss of your own freedom, your sleep patterns, and even your energy. The normality of your everyday life is gone and will not return to the way it was before you became a caregiver.

Additionally, you are continually facing the reality that you are caring for someone who has a disease with no cure. No matter how much you attempt to prepare mentally and emotionally for the day your loved one takes his or her last breath, when that day finally comes, you will most likely find that you were not as prepared as you thought. The grieving process may begin all over again. You will adjust to life without your loved one and assume a new role, and so will your family, as everyone tries to find his or her new place.

You may experience conflicting emotions, such as relief, regret, guilt, and sorrow. You may feel fear, anger, and bitterness and become withdrawn because you think that no one will understand or because you do not want to show or release your emotions in front of anyone. You may think you need to be strong for those around you—and to pretend that everything is ok.

What is grief? "Grief is the conflicting feelings caused by the end of or change in a familiar pattern of behavior." Thus, any changes in relationships with people, places, or events can cause the feeling we call grief. The range of emotions associated with grief varies greatly among different people and in the same person at different times.

If you are caring for someone with dementia, you are continually losing pieces of your loved one or client. Each of these specific losses can cause grief, which comes in three phases.

1. *Unfolding grief.* This grief comes as you experience many incremental losses caused by the effects of the dementia on the person. In some cases the dementia may progress rapidly, but more often than not, the losses occur over a long period of time. Not only are you slowly losing a parent, a spouse, or a friend; you are also losing the role that you have cherished as a daughter, son, wife, husband, relative, or friend along with the relationship that you had prior to the dementia. You may have lost the spouse who took care of the household finances, or the mother who loved to shop for clothes with you, or the father with whom you would spend Sundays working on the car or a project around the house.

2. *Anticipatory grief.* A caregiver experiences anticipatory grief with every passing day, knowing that there is an inevitable death ahead. Sometimes there is deep regret stemming from the fact that no matter how well you care for your loved one or client, he or she is facing the sunset of his or her life. It is very normal to experience regret and guilt not only when you wish that this person could be relieved of his or her suffering but also when you have the expectation of someday being released from your role as the care provider.

3. *Acute grief.* It can be agonizing to watch the dying process as the body shuts down. Acute grief comes as the physical death takes place and you face the finality that your loved one is gone. A combination of guilt and relief comes from both anticipatory and acute grief. The situation is often compounded by painful emotions and the losses of the caregiver's role and sense of identity.

During a grief seminar taught by Denise, I learned about these three phases of grief from a caregiver who also attended the seminar. This wonderful and sensitive man had lost his father to Alzheimer's just two weeks earlier. He had been his father's sole care provider for several years.

He shared with us the unfolding grief he felt as he lost precious parts of his father: his father's ability to care for his own bodily needs, his father's ability to care for his own finances, and his father's role as the father to his only son. He explained that even though he knew his father was declining physically and mentally with a terminal diagnosis of Alzheimer's, he dreaded the reality that his father would soon be gone altogether. Though he had attempted to brace himself for his father's death, he nevertheless felt extreme loss and emotional pain when his father passed away.

He even felt lost himself, since his whole routine and identity abruptly changed. Without his role as caregiver and the lifestyle he had gotten used to, he was no longer sure who he was and what his purpose was. While he had been caring for his father twenty-four hours a day, seven days a week, he had become fairly isolated and had only a few remaining friends. This gentleman was very appreciative of the grief seminar, as he felt Denise understood the conflicting emotions he was experiencing. This understanding helped him to look forward and not backward.

Perceptions and Approaches

Understanding and accepting the grief process guides you through acknowledging the loss. You can then give yourself permission to feel the emotions and will be aware that grief is a normal and natural part of the human experience. Among the feelings you may experience are the following:

- After a loss you may feel uncomfortable and may be afraid to show joy because it seems dishonoring to the person you have lost or because you are worried how others will perceive you if you do not behave in the way that you think they might expect you to behave.
- You might feel bad because, deep down, you are relieved that you are now finished with a very frustrating and unhappy role into which you were thrust.
- You might also feel that the caregiving was very rewarding and gave you unexpected closeness and treasured time with your loved one. Now that he or she is gone, you may feel empty.

Other people may want you to "get over it," "move on," or "be thankful that your loved one is in a better place," and they may assure you that "time heals." There will be days when you feel like avoiding contact with other people just so you will not have to hear anyone say anything trite. Outsiders believe these statements will help us work through the grief.

Denise and I and other caregivers who are experienced in the grief process understand that you would love to move on, if only you knew how. Many caregivers who share their own grief journeys candidly explain that the pain decreases but the void does not go away. One perception that may be helpful is to view the loss as a fork in the road on your journey. As you would do if you unexpectedly encountered a detour, you will find it beneficial to consult with others, look at a map, and have the right preparations to reach your destination. If you stay isolated and do not reach out to learn the tools you need to get you through the grieving process, the isolation could consume you, and this would not make the situation better.

An experienced grief counselor will help you to lean into the grief and will offer suggestions about how you can cope with the myriad complex feelings. A grief support group can also give you emotional support and the chance to interact with others who may be feeling similar emotions as they process their experiences. Getting support at this time will help you to understand how to rediscover the normality of everyday life and will assist you in transitioning to your new identity and purpose. I have found that grief counseling has also proven very helpful for caregivers.

To find a certified grief recovery specialist in your area, you can e-mail Denise Pedersen (griefandbeyond@gmail.com) or call the Grief Recovery Institute: 1-818-907-9600. A book on the subject of grief that I recommend is *The Grief Recovery Handbook*, by John W. James and Russell Friedman.

No matter where you are in the grieving process, trust your own journey. Let yourself explore and experience everything that grieving brings you. Look for support from trusted family, friends, and professionals who will help you continue going forward.

Above all, know that you need to choose the pace and the path that is right for you. Be gentle with yourself. You are a caregiver hero, and you may find that sharing your story will help others who follow behind you on the dementia caregiving journey.

Poetry, music, literature, and art can inspire us and soothe us as we grieve and as we cherish the lives of those we have lost. This excerpt from the song "Celebrate the Children," by Alan Pedersen, is one example that I treasure.

> We got to know the magic of their smiles, if only for a while,
> Wasn't it beautiful?
> They taught us how to love so deep, feel so complete,
> Wasn't it wonderful?
> Even if we knew that it would end,

If we had the chance we'd do it all again.

.   .   .   .

They left so many gifts behind for each of us to find,
It's magical!
They're with us every day, give help along the way,
It's spiritual!
They're part of everything we say and do,
We're better people now because of them, it's true.

CHAPTER NINETEEN

Lessons, Perceptions, and Approaches

A Reader's Guide

The dementia disease process will continually throw you curve balls. It never rests. As you encounter new challenges, the chapters in this book may take on a different meaning. Because every dementia journey is unique, you will need to remain adaptable throughout the entire experience. You may need to reread chapters in this book as you gain new insights over the course of your journey.

I wrote this book to help shift the process of caring for the person who has dementia from a burden into a meaningful experience. Whether you are an at-home family caregiver, a professional, or a family member or friend who is deeply involved in the care of someone who is residing in assisted living or in a skilled nursing home, you can use this book as a reference throughout the caregiving journey.

This final chapter summarizes the lessons, perceptions, and approaches offered by the stories in each of the previous chapters. The summaries may serve as reminders; you may also want to turn (or return) to a chapter that shares suggestions that may be particularly meaningful or helpful right now.

Chapter 1. Introduction: Navigating the Journey

You are the most important person in the caregiving process, and if you do not take care of yourself, you will not be able to provide care for your loved one or client. Sometimes you can only see one part of the dementia "elephant," but with an open mind you can continually "feel your way" through the caregiving process. I encourage you to access resources so that you can find the support you need. Every day, successful caregiving hinges on communicating with the person who has dementia. This chapter introduces the affirmative response method of communication, which will allow you to bridge the gap between you and the person with dementia.

Chapter 2. Peggy: The Ultimate Toll

Peggy's story is a poignant reminder of how caregivers strive to care for their loved ones on their own and often refuse to ask for help, even at the expense of their own lives.

Lessons learned. By taking care of yourself, you will give yourself the health and energy needed to take care of your loved one or client.

Perceptions and approaches. Adults with dementia base much of their communication on emotions. Listen to them carefully and speak from your heart.

Chapter 3. Deborah: A Daughter's Journey

Denial can make dementia more difficult to treat and can have consequences on overall quality of life—for both the person with dementia and you, the caregiver. Because no one wants to watch loved ones exhibit permanent and progressive loss of normal brain function, dementia caregivers are vulnerable to dementia-denial. Though this denial is based in self-protection, it ironically ends up making life more difficult for the caregiver and the person with dementia.

Lessons learned. Dementia-denial prevents people from seeking appropriate treatment and taking steps to better manage dementia symptoms. It allows abnormal behaviors to continue unchecked, with the possibility that someone may be injured. The antidote for dementia-denial is to become dementia-aware. The higher your level of knowledge about dementia early on during the care journey, the more aware and effective you will be as a caregiver.

Perceptions and approaches. To become a dementia-aware caregiver, you must reach out to and learn from resources in the medical community, remaining open to ongoing education about the many layers and constantly changing aspects of the dementia journey. Consider the bigger picture of how dementia dramatically affects more than just you and the one for whom you are caring. Most importantly, reach out to family, friends, and professionals for continuing support and assistance.

Chapter 4. Charles: There Is Nothing Wrong with Me

Some people with dementia will experience precisely the same kind of dementia-denial their caregivers exhibit. In both instances the denial is coming from the understandable desire to convince ourselves that everything is fine. However, *denial in the form of anosognosia is a far-reaching lack of awareness of impairment, causing most people not even to know they are ill.* Anosognosia *affects a substantial percentage of people with dementia, as well as those who have suffered strokes.*

Lessons learned. Because people with dementia who also have anosognosia may be entirely unaware of their impairments, they will often react with anger and defensiveness if confronted about their condition. For instance, they may firmly insist they do not have a problem and they may resist seeking medical help. Naturally, the family member or professional caregiver who has to deal with this problem can become exasperated and depleted.

Perceptions and approaches. Whether your loved one is in simple denial or has anosognosia, the most effective caregiving strategy is one of acceptance and empathy toward the symptoms and subsequent behaviors, rather than endlessly trying (and failing) to correct and confront the person about his or her dementia. Through strategies such as using positive action statements in communication, avoiding fact- and reason-based discussions that could lead to conflict, and taking good care of yourself, you will be much more successful in caring for your loved one.

Chapter 5. Frances: What Is Dementia?

This chapter addresses fundamental questions: what is dementia, and what are its causes and effects? It also emphasizes the need for caregivers to take care of themselves.

Lessons learned. Dementia is a symptom with many possible causes, such as Alzheimer's disease, Parkinson's disease, and stroke. It commonly manifests itself in behaviors like confusion, disorientation, repetitive behaviors, difficulty tracking or processing information, anxiety, fear, paranoia, and, most often, progressive short-term memory loss.

Perceptions and approaches. To understand how dementia affects people's memory, visualize the person you are caring for as a big 3-D jigsaw puzzle. The dementia progressively removes pieces of the puzzle, leaving an increasingly incomplete picture.

Chapter 6. Jill: Into the Dementia Wonderland

Although your loved one or client's memories may be fading, it is still possible to share meaningful moments with him or her. The story of Jill provides a deeper understanding of the wonderland in which the person who has dementia lives.

Lessons learned. To connect with the person who has dementia, you must enter that person's world, not attempt to bring him or her into your reality. The feelings remain long after the event has been forgotten.

Perceptions and approaches. It is important to remain calm as you provide care for the person who has dementia. The affirmative response method is the key to successful communication.

Chapter 7. Natalie: Much More than Words

This candid chapter explains that communication, especially when it comes to connecting with the person with dementia, is largely composed of nonverbal signals and cues.

Lessons learned. Communicating with a person who has dementia has less to do with your words than it has to do with the feelings you project. Pay close attention to your own stress level and the nonverbal signals you send.

Perceptions and approaches. You have the power to set the tone for each day by monitoring the feelings you bring into the relationship.

Chapter 8. Vada: Past, Present, and Future

Vada's story is a revealing example of how people with dementia can become stuck in negative past memories and how these memories become part of their ongoing present-time reality.

Lessons learned. While persons with dementia may become trapped in painful memories, allowing them to share those emotions will help them to move forward and find resolution.

Perceptions and approaches. When interacting with your client or loved one, develop a trusting relationship and provide a dignified and respectful atmosphere.

Chapter 9. Joe: Communicating the Gift of Value

Joe's story is an important reminder that everyone needs a sense of purpose and self-worth. Helping promote a loved one or client's feeling of significance is an integral part of improving the caregiving relationship.

Lessons learned. The person who has dementia will try to access feelings from past memories that give him or her a sense of value, joy, and security.

Perceptions and approaches. Using the affirmative response method, reaffirm the feelings and language from the person's past as if they were happening now.

Chapter 10. Lucy and Betty: Thinking Outside the Box

Through two different stories this chapter introduces the concept of creative interventions, which are uniquely tailored techniques to foster cooperation in difficult situations.

Lessons learned. Over time, dementia affects the person's abilities.

Learning about these changes allows you to have realistic expectations of what tasks the person can process and handle.

Perceptions and approaches. Practice patience. Encourage the person who has dementia to continue doing whatever he or she is still able to do. Celebrate the simplest and smallest accomplishments.

Chapter 11. Edna: You're Just Imagining Things

Unfortunately, as individuals struggle to cope with dementia, they often develop paranoia, including misperceptions or hallucinations about family members, old friends, and even strangers.

Lessons learned. Practicing new ways of reacting to these behaviors will give you the coping skills necessary to help manage them, thus giving you the key to making the person feel safe and supported.

Perceptions and approaches. No matter how outlandish the claim or accusation, listen and proceed as though you believe everything the person who has dementia is saying. Plan to take action that will give them a sense of relief. To them, the most frustrating response is for you to argue or to try to convince them that the situation is not real.

Chapter 12. Margie: If You Keep Doing What You Are Doing . . .

This chapter teaches how to apply the affirmative response method of communication through flexible approaches and creative thinking.

Lessons learned. You will never win an argument with someone who has dementia. If you are not receiving the desired affirmative response from your loved one or client, try a different approach.

Perceptions and approaches. Modify the environment, modify the behavior, and medicate as a last resort. (Always seek professional advice from the physician of the person you are caring for before making *any* changes in medication.)

Chapter 13. Harry: It's Bath Night!

The task of providing personal care, such as bathing and grooming, to the person who has dementia is frequently very difficult. This chapter presents helpful, straightforward suggestions on how to handle these challenges and how to cultivate more cooperative, peaceful interactions with care recipients.

Lessons learned. People with dementia tend to seek memories that make them feel safe and secure, but because of past memories, they may be resistant to allowing you to provide personal care.

Perceptions and approaches. With safety and comfort in mind, use an approach that may be familiar to your loved one or client through past experiences.

Chapter 14. Susan: Dealing with Disruption

Dementia can devastatingly disrupt individual lives and those of entire families. Susan's story powerfully illustrates the need to access supportive community resources.

Lessons learned. Caregivers often struggle with the overwhelming juggling act of raising children, maintaining a full-time career, and providing care for aging loved ones or clients.

Perceptions and approaches. Never be afraid to ask for help. Asking for help is a necessary part of the caregiving role. Educate yourself and utilize all your options.

Chapter 15. Grace: Moving beyond Guilt

Many caregivers feel guilty because they are not able to manage all of the caregiving responsibilities on their own. Grace's story demonstrates how to escape the burden of unnecessary guilt that makes so many caregivers avoid requesting help. Asking for assistance opens the door to relief.

Lessons learned. Guilt is an extremely common emotion that prevents caregivers from acknowledging the need to take care of themselves.

Perceptions and approaches. Learning about guilt and what may be causing you to feel guilty will help you move past it.

Chapter 16. Virginia: Laughter Is Therapeutic

Sometimes the old clichés are true: laughter is wonderful medicine. Virginia's experience provides an example of how to see the humor in even the most trying situations.

Lessons learned. Laughter is one of the best stress-busters available.

Perceptions and approaches. Look for different opportunities to bring laughter into your life. This can be done daily!

Chapter 17. Beatrice and Henry: The Power of Gratitude

Having a sense of gratitude in a caregiving role is challenging but essential. Gratitude can help make the entire caregiving journey far more fulfilling.

Lessons learned. By changing your perspective and focusing on the positive instead of the negative, you will be able to see things more clearly and better understand the importance of the moments shared with others.

Perceptions and approaches. Take the time to keep a journal of the good things and experiences you have in your life, no matter how small they may seem at the time.

Chapter 18. Sean: The Puzzling Pieces of Grief

When we experience a tragedy, grief will inevitably follow. As we care for someone with dementia, we experience grief in multiple stages.

Lessons learned. If you are caring for someone with dementia, you are slowly losing pieces of your loved one as the disease progresses. It is normal and natural to experience grief every time these losses occur. In spite of the grief, you are not broken and you do not need to be fixed.

Perceptions and approaches. Through every phase of the grieving process, it is important to let yourself feel the pain and conflicting emotions. Find someone who will listen to you without criticizing you. You must allow yourself to travel down your own unique grieving path.

The Dementia-Aware Guide to Caregiving

Practice putting these newfound lessons to use with this dementia-aware guide, which follows this chapter.

Caregivers from all walks of life, professions, and backgrounds need others to support them throughout the process of caring for a person with dementia. In America, there are millions of caregivers like you who face the difficult job of caring for an adult with cognitive impairment. My goal is to extend my supportive hands through this book and remind you that you are not alone. Keep this book close by in the coming days and months so you can find the information most relevant to your situation on a daily or hourly basis. You might also want to pass this book along to others who may be entering into the caregiving journey.

I am here to support you, and if you wish to contact me, you can e-mail me directly at help@laurawayman.com or www.laurawayman .com. Although caregiving can often be a thankless behind-the-scenes job, you are of great value. I honor and admire you, and I look forward to hearing from you.

The Dementia-Aware Guide to Caregiving

Congratulations! You are now well on the road toward becoming a dementia-aware caregiver. Every dementia care journey is unique—and you can also expect that the landscape will be constantly changing. Whether you are a family caregiver or a professional caregiver, it is important to remain adaptable with your care approach so you can successfully manage the dementia-related symptoms and behaviors in the moment.

Even with all of the lessons offered in this book, you may still have reservations about how to be a dementia-aware caregiver on a day-to-day basis. While it is important to individualize care approaches to the singular circumstances presented, there are many common challenges associated with dementia. To support you with caring for your loved one, client, or resident, this Dementia-Aware Guide to Caregiving is a quick reference tool for responding to difficult behaviors, as well as a way to practice this essential change in your care approach. As you read the examples below, begin to evaluate each challenge and consider options to put into practice for your individualized dementia-aware care approach. Then as you read the successful dementia-aware care approach these caregivers chose, reflect on whether your care approach choice was similar. You can even go a step further and think of other options, or a combination of options, that might also provide successful care outcomes.

Here is a "dementia reality mantra" that is useful to many people: "*I cannot stop, change, or fix the dementia symptoms or behaviors. Instead, I can only manage them.*" As you begin each day in your caregiving role, it is valuable to be mindful of this mantra. You may even want to recite it out loud.

Practice and utilize the tools in this Dementia-Aware Guide to Caregiving so you may enjoy more positive and loving care outcomes. I want to take this opportunity to remind you that you are doing a great job! Keep up the good work! You make a difference!

Challenges with Personal Hygiene

Getting dressed, taking a shower, and brushing teeth can be very complex tasks for a person living with dementia because of the many steps involved. For individuals with dementia, this process is laden with too much information. Another obstacle is that some people with dementia may have an altered sense of hot and cold, since the disease has damaged the region of their brains that controls their internal thermostats. They may even feel abnormal sensations from the water itself. This adds another layer of complexity to bathing and showering. All of these factors make maintaining personal hygiene a significant obstacle for some caregivers.

Strategies

- Offer the person limited choices and do not ask questions. For example, you can say "It is time to take a bath" or "Come with me."
- Break down the tasks into simple steps and calmly and patiently explain each step, using easy-to-understand directions and respectful, affirming language. "Lift up your arms." "Let's put on this shirt." "You look nice!"
- Encourage the person to do as much as possible on his or her own, whether brushing teeth or using soap and a washcloth.
- Lay out the soap, washcloth, towel, and clean clothes in se-

quence so the person with dementia can participate in each
step in the task.

- When assisting with showering or bathing, use reassuring
language like "This water feels good." Let the person touch
the water before getting into the bath or shower. Sometimes
gently pouring water over the person's hands will help him
or her relax. Or start with a basic "foot soak" and work your
way up.
- Honor the person's sense of modesty—use a towel to cover
sensitive areas while you assist with the washing of arms,
legs, and back, or allow the person to remain partially
dressed during the process.
- Accept that there will be good days and bad days. If you are
encountering extreme resistance that could escalate into a
worse situation, let the task go. Try again when the person
appears calmer and more receptive, perhaps the next
morning or before bed.

A dementia-aware caregiver will evaluate what the person is feeling.

- ➤ Listen to what the person is saying—not just the words, but
observe his or her facial expressions and actions.
- ➤ Smile, breathe and relax—your calmness will comfort the
person and reduce agitation.

Scenario

"I just took a shower this morning! I am not dirty!" Harvey
would insist to his wife, Sara, whenever she would ask him to
take a shower. This dialogue would go on and on, spiralling
into a full-blown argument as Sara attempted to reason with
her once fastidious husband, telling him he had not showered
in many days and trying to convince him that his hair was
dirty and his clothes smelly and stained. Asking Harvey to
make these choices and process the truth about his unhygienic
condition was cognitively overwhelming and only persisted in
making this undertaking miserable for both of them.

The Successful Dementia-Aware Approach

Sara decided to try changing her care approach. Instead of asking Harvey if he wanted to take a shower, or giving him options about when he needed to shower as she had in the past, she instead just led him to the bathroom that she had prepared in advance, making him less apprehensive and resistant. The idea is not to do a surprise attack but instead to minimize hesitation caused by "information overload." Sara learned that when she "thinks" for Harvey and remains calm, confident, and in the moment, he has less time to resist and feel anxious about what the showering event is all about. She also chooses her battles and changes her strategies according to how Harvey is feeling. Harvey still resists sometimes even with the transformed care approach, and on those days Sara chooses to use her time for other tasks and let this one go until later, or even to wait a day or two.

The Frustration of Negative Responses

One of the most common frustrations among caregivers is the propensity for people with dementia to say, "No!" Caregivers cannot understand why their loved ones so often refuse to do the very things they have done willingly and eagerly in the past. The reasons are actually pretty straightforward. Dementia impacts memory, processing information, reasoning, and language, so it is difficult for individuals with dementia to understand what others ask of them. They also often lose their ability to express what they are feeling, and the outward behavior becomes a means of communication. If they feel reluctant, afraid, or confused, they react exactly how most people would in situations that make them feel uncomfortable: "No—go away!" And if the caregiver inadvertently continues to share too much information, the behavior may escalate from saying "No" to saying mean, inappropriate, or even hurtful things.

Strategies

- Respond to the emotion, not the behavior, and attempt to direct the individual toward feelings of calmness. For example, if the person appears nervous and refuses to come with you, do not directly attempt to change his or her mind. Instead, you can say things like "It's such a beautiful day today" or "It's been a long time since the weather has been this nice—we should go outside and enjoy it."
- Avoid trying to reason with your loved one and do not attempt to explain the request in detail, since he or she may not be able to follow lengthy explanations.
- Share less information. Phrase your instructions in the form of gentle directive statements, rather than questions, options, or facts and figures (such as how many days it's been since you last took a walk).
- Instead of asking the person if she or he wants to go for a drive in the country, simply say: "Let's go for a drive."

A dementia-aware caregiver chooses the battle and changes the strategy as needed.

- ➤ Do not try to correct behaviors that do not pose an immediate safety issue to you or the person with dementia.
- ➤ While remaining calm and providing reassurance, redirect the person with dementia by taking his or her attention off the situation that is causing anxiety.
- ➤ Remain fluid and flexible, adjusting to the person's behaviors as needed.

Scenario

David was a loving and dedicated caregiver for his wife, Mabel. They had enjoyed a devoted married life together for sixty years, rarely ever being away from each other for more than a day or two. Seven years ago, Mabel was diagnosed with Alzheimer's disease after her dementia symptoms worsened for several years. For most of her life, Mabel was a soft-spoken and polite lady, and David had often expressed admiration for how she always seemed to know the right thing to say. That is why it was so disheartening when Mabel began at first responding with a resounding "No" when asked most questions, then progressed to cursing under her breath, and later started hurling a host of swear words that surprised all who knew her. This was most evident, and getting steadily worse, when David would ask if she was hungry. The reaction would be even more heightened if he tacked on more complex options, such as what she wanted for dinner, if she wanted to go out to one of her favorite restaurants, and what time she would like eat. As the questions continued she would become more and more agitated and the "sailor-talk" would progress to mean, hurtful, and inappropriate rages at David in private and out in public. David would apologize for her, but he remained confused about her reaction. "I am gentle and don't deny her anything. I just want to ask her what she wants. She makes up things and says the most horrible things to me—words I never knew she had ever heard!"

The Successful Dementia-Aware Approach

David attended one of my trainings and listened intently about addressing the underlying emotions, reacting with calm indifference to the behavior, and practicing less talking and more doing. The trigger for Mabel's fearful, angry, and anxious feelings was his unrealistic expectation that she could still process his questions or other details about dinner: restaurants, time to eat, where to eat, what to eat, getting in and out of the car, reading a menu, and so on. This information, familiar to her in the past, now just made her feel nervous, agitated, and put on the spot about giving the "correct" response. David realized that it was much kinder and calming for them both if he simply chose to give her only the information she could manage in the moment. He also recognized that going out to a restaurant was far too overwhelming; Mabel was much more at ease just having her meal placed in front of her without the before-meal discussions, requests for her input, or conversations concerning her feelings.

Refusing to Go to the Doctor

No one wants to hear that he or she has dementia. It can take supportiveness, tact, and creativity to encourage someone to have a physician check about worrisome symptoms. Understandably, such evaluations tend to produce anxiety. Additionally, people with dementia—and possibly suffering from denial in the form of anosognosia—may not be aware of the loss of normal brain function. Because they feel fine, they can't imagine why they would need to see a physician.

Strategies

- To "sell" the doctor's visit to the individual with dementia, use another health complaint (e.g., arthritis or a heart check) as a reason for making a doctor's appointment.
- Another option is to make it *your* issue, rather than his or her issue. Explain that you want to talk to the doctor about your own recent memory challenges and would like your loved one to come with you for support.
- Solicit the help of a trusted "third party," someone other than a family member, to suggest, for example, that regular checkups are important for everyone.
- Call or e-mail the doctor in advance of a routine checkup to express concerns and ask about a dementia screening.
- Provide the doctor's office with a list of symptoms and changes you have observed (dates and times of incidents) to indicate a pattern. This way, you will not have to share these details in front of the person during the visit.
- Keep it positive. Do not focus on the person's deficits but rather on his or her retained skills and strengths.
- Acknowledge fear or other emotions: "It's not pleasant to think

about, and I can only imagine how this makes you feel. Let's find out what is going on together."

- Just be there—your presence can be very calming and comforting, such as an arm around the shoulder or holding hands.

*A **dementia-aware caregiver** does not attempt to win an argument with someone who has dementia.*

➤ Do not expect the person with dementia to comply with a doctor's orders, prescriptions, or recommended care options.
➤ It is kinder for you to make decisions that are in his or her best interests.

Scenario

The whispered conversations among the siblings about Dad were becoming more prevalent. The oldest daughter living nearby was the first to notice the changes in Dad, and then finally her sister and two brothers living miles away agreed they could not stay in dementia-denial any longer. Dad was mixing up his grandchildren's names, had several minor scratches and dents that became visible on his car without explanation, and showed up for a family event on the wrong day. The family sat down with Dad and insisted he go to the doctor to get checked out. Dad flatly denied there was a problem. He blamed the car damage on other "bad drivers"; he claimed the date mix-up resulted from several family members "having given him conflicting dates"; and he maintained that his confusion with names was simply a matter of the family "mishearing his responses." Reasoning or badgering from the adult children only led to more resistance, so they decided to come together and change the way they were communicating with Dad about the situation.

The Successful Dementia-Aware Approach

The family decided to try a "third party approach." Since Dad was not willing to listen to them, they asked the pastor of Dad's church to suggest that he might want to see his doctor, as everyone over 60 should get their heart and blood sugar tested regularly. The pastor mentioned that he himself was making an appointment to check his own health. This worked like a charm, as Dad was more apt to listen to someone other than the adult children. By choosing to ask this influential and trusted non–family member to take the message to Dad and reassuring him it was a customary undertaking for someone his age, as well as wisely avoiding the sensitive subject concerning his self-disclaimed dementia symptoms, the mission of getting Dad to the doctor was accomplished.

Confusion and Agitation Caused by Transition Trauma

"I want to go home!" "This isn't my house!" "When are we leaving?" "Why are we here?" Wanting to go home is one of the most common reactions for people with dementia who have relocated to unfamiliar environments, such as a different home or a memory care facility. This is often referred to as *transition trauma*. Transition trauma is a term used to describe the stress that a person with dementia may experience when changing living environments. The length of time and severity of the transition trauma is quite individual and is usually temporary. It is relieved as the individual builds friendships, gains trust, and develops a sense of purpose and belonging in his or her new community.

Often, individuals in a new environment are trying to feel connected to a place where they felt safe and had more control in their lives. Instead of trying to convince people with dementia they are "home," respond to the immediate need, which is to make them feel safe and secure.

Caregivers may feel guilty over recent moves or placements of their loved ones and feel obligated to provide detailed justifications of why they made these decisions: "Remember—you had a fall and lay on the floor and got dehydrated, and the doctor said it's not safe for you to live alone anymore. So we found this place! And I know it will take some time to adjust, but this is really the best thing for you, since it's not an option to go back home." However, lengthy explanations are beyond what people with dementia can process. The likely result will be negative reactions and agitation. Inevitably things will get worse with that approach.

Strategies

- Give the person the opportunity to experience a different environment and "go out," such as to a secure courtyard at the facility or a pretty walking path in the local neighborhood.
- If the person asks specific questions—like "When are we leaving?"—try responses such as: "We can leave later—right now the traffic is terrible." "The forecast is calling for bad weather." "It's too late to leave tonight."
- Say as little as possible about the behaviors associated with the request to "go home." For example, if the person has packed all of his or her belongings in a suitcase and is demanding to leave, redirect the person by finding another activity, listening to music, or getting a snack.
- Figure out what actions and simple statements are going to make the person feel the safest in the moment, yet accept that he or she may feel the same way and want to "go home" again a little while later.
- Repeat whatever actions or statements work. If agitation increases, make a note of it so you can coach other caregivers or family members about what seems to work versus what does not.
- Talk about a special memory associated with what "home" represents to the person—a family pet, a favorite meal— and then bring up relatable examples from your own life and use them to redirect the conversation. "You had a pet cat? I love cats too! Our cat had a bunch of kittens . . ."

- It may be necessary to access more assistance during the peak time the person is experiencing transition trauma. Consider hiring a caregiver from an outside agency temporarily while the person is adjusting to give the one-on-one support and companionship above and beyond what the care community's staff can provide.

A dementia-aware caregiver understands that every person wants to feel safe and comfortable.

➤ The better you know the person with dementia, the more easily you can read his or her emotions and find a way to create a sense of familiarity and security.

Scenario

Our family had opted for out-of-home placement when my grandfather's dementia symptoms had become too stressful for our grandmother to manage at home. As my grandfather's Alzheimer's progressed, he would sit and gaze quietly and for long periods out the window of the memory care facility throughout most of our visit. Then at some point during many of these visits, Grandfather would become agitated, turn his gaze to us, and say loudly with great concern: "Are you taking me home now? I am ready to go home, get me out of here!" This would be followed by extreme agitation and impatience when we would not immediately produce the car and take him home. At first we would all freeze, not sure what to say or do. We were afraid that if we used any of our previously unsuccessful attempts to reassure him that he was "home" or that he needed to stay here due to his dementia, the result would ultimately be more anger and frustration. It was obvious that our trying to reason with or change his yearning to go home would only perpetuate his unaddressed feelings of loneliness, abandonment, and distress.

The Successful Dementia-Aware Approach

Then one day we were treated to a demonstration of a true dementia-aware care approach by one of the professional caregivers on staff. Instead of trying to talk Grandfather out of his longing to reach "home," this brilliant caregiver knew to simply skip any attempt to orient him to our reality and instead *hear* what he meant by the word "home." It was a feeling, not a place, and the caregiver knew she could help him experience these feelings of "home" right there in the moment. By directly talking to his feelings she could meet his emotional needs by saying: "Come listen to the music first. We both enjoy the music so much." Then as she confidently smiled and took Grandfather's hand he happily followed her down the hall to the music activity without a second look our way. From that day on we changed our visits to ones that included sharing special memories that allowed him to experience more moments of comfort, security, and love.

Difficulty with New or Changing Routines

Although people with dementia typically lose recent memories, everyday routines are part of a different memory structure in the brain that tends to remain intact longer. By sticking to the same daily routines, individuals with dementia are less likely to become frustrated about trying to decide what to do next. Elements of a routine may include eating breakfast before getting dressed, sitting in the same recliner in the living room each morning and watching television, attending to personal care in the afternoon, taking a walk, having a scoop of ice cream, or taking a bath in the evening. While the order of these daily activities may seem insignificant, they provide a sense of familiarity and purpose. Caregivers have the opportunity to create stability by helping people with dementia maintain their routines.

Strategies

- If you are a family caregiver, you know your loved one's daily rituals better than anyone else, so you are in a unique position to customize and refine his or her routine so it includes meaningful activities. Be sure to share this individualized knowledge about your loved one's wishes as you reach out for additional help from professionals providing in-home care, assisted living / memory care, or adult day care.
- Leave recognizable furniture and artwork in the same places they have always been, unless they could pose safety hazards.
- If the person with dementia has moved to an assisted living or memory care facility, recreate the home-like environment in his or her room or apartment as closely as possible—though simplifying is the best route. If the previous environment was cluttered, choose to use the most obviously recognizable and cherished pieces (for example, that recliner chair for watching TV) and de-clutter as much as possible.
- Allow the person to participate in his or her routine tasks for as long as he or she is able—it may not be perfect and a given task could take three times longer, but maintaining independence promotes dignity and reduces physical strain on the caregiver.
- Adjust your expectations as the disease advances. It is up to the caregiver to decide what activities are still reasonable and safe for the individual with dementia to perform and which activities the person needs help doing.

A dementia-aware caregiver uses routine as a tool.

- ➤ Organizing your own day may take little conscious effort, but giving structure to the day of a person with dementia may pose special challenges.
- ➤ By allowing the person with dementia to stick to his or her routines, you also save yourself from having to think too much about how to organize his or her day.

Scenario

When I first took on the care of my aunt, who has Parkinson's dementia, I stumbled often, having to figure out through trial and error the best ways to manage her individual dementia symptoms. One of the most crucial things I learned early on was that routine was very important to her. Even relatively small things that I considered insignificant would often still be of great consequence to her. Aunt Beverly moved into her own small house on our property, and as I spent more time caring for her I found my caregiving role was much less stressful if I kept her things in the same place and her day on a strict routine. And this not only made my job easier, it also helped Aunt Beverly to feel more calm, safe, and confident. This was very evident on the first Christmas my aunt spent with us, when I had not yet seen how upsetting holidays may be to someone with dementia. Naturally, my other family members and I wanted to celebrate as we always had before Aunt Beverly came to stay with me, but we did not yet know how important it would be to keep changes for her to the bare minimum. The week of Christmas brought about many routine changes such as out-of-town visitors arriving at her usual bedtime or meal time, or a visit interrupting her favorite television show. There was even a change in environment, Aunt Beverly had to come the short distance to our home for the big Christmas dinner and she was completely disoriented with all of the changes in her surroundings, together with a stream of new names and faces, ongoing noise, conversation, and delayed meal times. These changes enjoyed by the other family members caused Aunt Beverly extreme anxiety and confusion that escalated to very unpleasant behaviors. She suddenly went from sweetly confused to restless and angry, demanding that all these "strangers" get out of her house. As the family members looked at her in shock I took her hand and gently led her back across the yard to her quiet and familiar little home.

The Successful Dementia-Aware Approach

After I got Aunt Beverly back to her own house, I stayed with her until she calmed down. As I reflected on the holiday festivities that I had mistakenly thought she would enjoy I realized this dramatic change in her routine was what was making her feel overwhelmed. As a result of this episode, I now bring meals at the same time, bring her pills at the same time, and set her television to the channel of her favorite shows at the same time each day. And I always put things in the same place: her pills, remote, slippers, shoes, and so on— even if it is a holiday. As I have become more dementia-aware I have come to realize that change is difficult for Aunt Beverly and that sticking to a structured schedule meets two objectives: relieving my caregiver stress and helping her to maintain her abilities and cope with her losses.

Making a Move

As the dementia causes progressive cognitive impairment and physical decline, it often becomes necessary for individuals to receive more appropriate levels of care outside of their homes. This can be a difficult decision for family caregivers to make, but it can also be in the best interests of both the caregivers and their loved ones. Family caregivers can sometimes lose sight of the fact that the demands of full-time caregiving are more than any one person can realistically manage. The decision to move loved ones to assisted living or memory care facilities can be based on a combination of factors, such as:

- The caregivers' health is being compromised (e.g., by sleep deprivation, caregivers' own physical limitations, and chronic medical conditions).
- The home environment is no longer safe or easy to navigate (e.g., because of the presence of stairs and narrow doorways).
- The individual who has dementia needs significant help with activities of daily living (eating, dressing, and personal hygiene).

- The care needs have increased significantly (e.g., as a result of incontinence, aggression, or wandering).

Strategies

- A successful move requires significant support from outside resources. Reach out to care professionals in the local community, such as a senior placement agency or the staff at an assisted living or memory care facility.
- To the degree that he or she is still able to participate in the decision-making process, the person with dementia should give input on the move. However, if anosognosia is a part of the dementia journey, it is crucial to share *less* information concerning their condition and any necessary care decisions.
- A senior placement agency or facility will complete a thorough intake and assessment, which involves meeting with you and other key family members, as well as with the person who has dementia, to evaluate his or her care needs.
- The assisted living or memory care facility should be staffed with professionals who are properly trained in dementia care and who will continue to work in collaboration with the family.
- Share your loved one's history with the facility staff, including his or her hobbies, favorite activities, likes and dislikes, passions, and pastimes. This helps the staff create an environment in which your loved one will thrive. It also empowers the staff to develop a personalized dementia-aware relationship with your loved one.

A dementia-aware caregiver prepares for the future and takes care of his or her own health, even if it means moving his or her loved one to an assisted living or memory care facility.

- ➢ Planning before the move will help make the transition as smooth as possible.
- ➢ Families that take the time to explore all their options are

better able to make an informed decision about the care setting.

➤ Placing your loved one in a facility does not minimize the importance of your caregiving role. You are simply inviting professionals to support your loved one's care needs while you continue to love and care for the person.

Scenario

I am the lone caregiver of my mother, 72, who has had Alzheimer's for the past seven years or so. My dad, who was her primary caregiver, passed away two years ago. Soon after I moved in to take over the caregiving role, I realized what an undertaking he had endured as the dementia worsened. They were married for fifty-two blissful years, and for most of those years they enjoyed reasonable health. Now, two years after I took over the caregiving role, Mom has declined significantly in her dementia. Her symptoms have gone beyond what I can take care of. I always feel so guilty when making care decisions for her, yet she is completely unable to make them for herself. She does not want to move out of her home and she wants me out of the house, as she feels she is perfectly able to care for herself. Unfortunately, due to the overwhelming stress of caring for Mom, I have lost twenty-five pounds and I look like I am the sick one. I have to constantly find ways of going around her resistance to get things done. I feel so frustrated and guilty that I needed to hire a professional in-home caregiver to sit with her while I run errands for three hours a day, and then all my mom does is complain that she doesn't need or want anyone in her home. I would love to access more in-home help and keep Mom in her home longer, but financially this is not feasible—nor would Mom go along with this approach, so there would be ongoing heated arguments. I love her so much but she is telling everyone in the world she does not want or need me here in spite of the lengths I have gone to help her. And I feel so guilty that at one time, before the dementia changed her, I had promised I would care for her in her home if Dad could not. I just did not understand that when I made that promise her dementia would later force me to amend such a naive yet heartfelt pledge.

The Successful Dementia-Aware Approach

After taking a step back and assessing Mom's mushrooming needs, as well as considering my own diminished health, I have come to the painful conclusion that, first, Mom's care has become too demanding for me to appropriately handle, and, second, it is not safe for her in the house as it is currently set up. To adequately keep her safe in her home now I would at the very least need to install special shower temperature controls, offer constant supervision when she is using the stairs, put together a danger-free kitchen, install keypad door locks, and provide nighttime awake care. Therefore, I feel it is important to access out-of-home care before it is too late or we are faced with a crisis such as a fall or her wandering off and getting lost. It's all so complicated—but I realize this will make us both better, and I do this out of love and concern. I will find her a memory care community that will partner with me to deliver the care, the love, the safe environment, and dignity she deserves.

By becoming increasingly dementia-aware you will experience more meaningful moments with your loved one and feel more confident and empowered in your individual care role. In the course of this journey you will develop a deeper understanding of the impact dementia has on individuals, their families, organizations, neighborhoods, and the world.

REFERENCES

Chapter 1, page 4: "My personal studies in this field have included excellent foundational resources"

Naomi Feil, *The Validation Breakthrough: Simple Techniques for Communicating with People with "Alzheimer's Type Dementia,"* 2nd ed. (Baltimore: Health Professions Press, 2002); Nancy L. Mace and Peter V. Rabins, *The 36-Hour Day: A Family Guide to Caring for People with Alzheimer Disease, Other Dementias, and Memory Loss in Later Life,* 5th ed. (Baltimore: Johns Hopkins University Press, 2011); Virginia Bell and David Troxel, *The Best Friend's Approach to Alzheimer's Care* (Baltimore: Health Professions Press, 1996).

Chapter 2, page 9: "Caring for a person with dementia is described by the National Family Caregivers Association as being three times more work"

National Family Caregivers Association, "Caregiving Statistics from the National Family Caregivers Association," www.nfcacares.org.

Chapter 4, page 22: "President Wilson 'would be seized with what, to a normal person, would seem to be inexplicable outbursts of emotion.'"

Errol Morris, "The Anosognosic's Dilemma: Something Wrong But You'll Never Know What It Is" (part three of a series), *New York Times* (June 22, 2010).

Chapter 4, page 23: "Our right brain is wired to detect anomalies and new information and incorporates these into our sense of reality"

Errol Morris, "The Anosognosic's Dilemma: Something Wrong But You'll Never Know What It Is" (part four of a series), *New York Times* (June 22, 2010).

Chapter 5, page 29: "Dementia is not a specific disease. It's an overall term that describes a wide range of symptoms associated with a decline in memory or other thinking skills severe enough to reduce a person's ability." http://www.alz.org/what-is-dementia.asp.

Chapter 5, page 29: "For example, an exposure to anesthesia increases the risk of dementia"

"Cognitive Problems Following Anesthesia," interview with Dr. Alex Bekker, *Alzheimer's Association Newsletter*, New York Chapter, 33 (Summer 2009): 53–54. Available at https://www.alznyc.org/nyc/newsletter/summer2009/37.asp.

Alex Bekker and Others, "Does Mild Cognitive Impairment Increase the Risk of Developing Postoperative Cognitive Dysfunction?" *Am J Surg* 199, no. 6 (June 2010): 782–88.

Chapter 5, page 30: "In addition, there is a difference between dementia and delirium."

Carla Marie Boulianne, "Elderly Dementia and Delirium: Causes of Elder Confusion Determine Treatments and Outcome," Suite101.com, June 15, 2008, http://seniors-health-medicare.suite101.com/article.cfm/elderly_dementia_and_delirium.

Chapter 5, page 30: "According to the *Merck Manual for Healthcare Professionals*"

Merck Manuals Online Medical Library, Section: Neurological Disorders, Subject: Delirium and Dementia, www.merck.com/mmpe/index.html.

Chapter 5, page 33: "Frances may also have been experiencing Capgras syndrome."

Named after Jean Marie Joseph Capgras, French psychiatrist, 1873–1950.

Chapter 7, page 47: "According to Albert Mehrabian"

A. Mehrabian, *Silent Messages* (Belmont, CA: Wadsworth, 1981; currently distributed by Albert Mehrabian).

Chapter 7, page 50: "According to the Family Caregiver Alliance" www.caregiver.org/caregiver-health.

Chapter 7, page 50: "A recent study by Kipps and others" C. M. Kipps et al., "Understanding Social Dysfunction in the Behavioural Variant of Frontotemporal Dementia: The Role of Emotion and Sarcasm Processing," *Brain: A Journal of Neurology* 132, no. 3 (2009): 592–603.

Chapter 11, page 75: "HeartMath training programs, coaching, publications, licensing programs, and innovative technology may help people live more rewarding and healthy lives—personally and professionally." www.heartmath.com/.

Chapter 11, page 75: "A program called Snoezelen Therapy" Jan Hulsegge and Ad Verheul, *Snoezelen: Another World* (Chesterfield, Derbyshire: Rompa, 1988). This program is also described at http://en.wikipedia.org/wiki/Snoezelen.

Chapter 12, page 80: "Research is showing that some relatively basic interventions that do not involve pharmaceuticals can be used" J. Cohen-Mansfield, A. Libin, and M. S. Marx, "Nonpharmacological Treatment of Agitation: A Controlled Trial of Systematic Individualized Intervention," *Journals of Gerontology Series A: Biological Sciences and Medical Sciences* 62 (2007): 908–17.

Chapter 13, page 90: "*Bathing without a Battle*" Ann Louise Barrick, Joanne Rader, Beverly Hoeffer, Philip D. Sloane, and Stacey Biddle, *Bathing without a Battle: Person-Directed Care of Individuals with Dementia*, 2nd ed. (New York: Springer, 2008).

Chapter 14, page 93: "Sixteen million Americans find themselves sandwiched between two generations" Todd C. Ratner, "Some Things to Chew On: Estate Planning Considerations for the Baby Boomer/Sandwich Generation," *Business to Business*, February 4, 2008, www.baconwilson.com/publications/articles.html.

Chapter 15, page 98: "As Dorothy Womack has written" Dorothy Womack, "Caregiver Guilt," *Today's Caregiver*, www.caregiver.com/articles/caregiver/caregiver_guilt.htm.

Chapter 16, page 100: "As comedian Bob Newhart reportedly said"
Bob Newhart, U.S. comedian and television actor (1929–) quoted in Laura Moncur's "Motivational Quotations," http://www.quotationspage.com/mqotd.html.

Chapter 17, page 103: "Research shows that caring for someone with dementia"
National Family Caregivers Association, "Caregiving Statistics from the National Family Caregivers Association," www.nfcacares.org.

Chapter 18, pages 109 and 112: "Grief is the conflicting feelings" and "A book on the subject of grief"
John W. James and Russell Friedman, *The Grief Recovery Handbook: The Action Program for Moving beyond Death, Divorce, and Other Losses* (New York: HarperCollins, 1998).

Chapter 18, page 112: "The song 'Celebrate the Children'"
"Celebrate the Children," lyrics by Alan Pedersen, www.everashley music.com. Reprinted with permission.

ABOUT THE AUTHORS

Laura Wayman

With over a decade of experience and a strong dedication to quality aging, Laura Wayman holds an associate's degree in gerontology and is a certified social services designee. Her innovative approach to the caregiving process has given her valuable insights into how caregivers can enhance and even enjoy their relationships with their loved ones or clients. During her career, she has developed the affirmative response method, an easy-to-learn, easy-to-apply communication style for connecting with the person who has dementia. As a result, she is a sought-after speaker with extensive experience in keynote addresses and break-out programs. Laura also teaches her "becoming dementia-aware" care approach and communication techniques at a local community college in northern California. She provides in-service training for assisted living, memory care, skilled nursing, and in-home professional caregivers on gentle and effective redirection tools and a communication approach that works. She is often invited to educate caregivers about how to become dementia-aware, helping them to learn effective techniques, and directing them to further dementia-aware community resources.

Contributing author Alicia Murray, B.A. Gerontology, M.A. Organizational Leadership, has hands-on experience in the assisted living and memory care field. She has done extensive research on the dementia caregiving industry, focusing on individualized plans that allow for all residents to experience homelike feelings of safety and security within the memory care setting. Alicia is able to identify and utilize flexible techniques with the goal of helping to maintain independence and quality of life during the progression of Alzheimer's disease and related dementias. Alicia encourages her care staff to facilitate creative activities, respecting the uniqueness of each community and individual. With her engaging approach, she helps caregivers learn to take better care of themselves while continuing to provide each resident with care in ways that can be both meaningful and enjoyable.

Contributing author Denise Pedersen is a certified grief recovery specialist. In 2004, as a result of having lost her oldest child, Sean, in an automobile accident, she founded the Sean Sullivan Project to reach out and help bereaved families in the Roseville/Sacramento, California, area. This project has become an important grief support group in the northern California area, and Denise has personally reached out to hundreds of hurting people after the loss of a child. In February 2010, Denise married Alan Pedersen, an award-winning songwriter, successful recording artist, and nationally recognized speaker on grief and loss. A few days later they began the Angels across the USA 2010 Tour (www.AngelsAcrosstheUSA.com, DenisePedersen2010@gmail .com), sponsored in part by bereaved families. The goal of this tour—with visits to more than 120 cities and at least one concert event in each of the forty-eight contiguous states—was to raise community awareness and draw media attention to local grief organizations that provide resources for the bereaved.

INDEX